Who Can Care For Me Now?

Elizabeth Orr

Clink Street
London | New York

Published by Clink Street Publishing 2018

Copyright © 2018

First edition.

ISBN:
978-1-912562-96-1- paperback
978-1-912562-97-8 - ebook

I dedicate this book to Norman who possibly would not have won "the best brother award" but he was "my" brother and that was good enough for me. Norm was an easy going chap who would not hurt a fly. Like so many others, he did not deserve to be subjected to so much suffering and to such an awful, prolonged, death.

I would also like to dedicate this book to:

- All those who have suffered from any form of brain disease/ illness and their family and friends
- Individuals living in a care home or nursing home who are unhappy
- All those navigating their way through the maze of systems/ procedures in an attempt to care for their family member or loved one.

Foreword

Elizabeth was recommended to us by an existing client during February 2015 as she was looking for advice and guidance with particular reference to the financial implications of caring for her brother. Norman, her brother, passed away May 2015 so by the time we met Elizabeth, she was already in the later stages of her challenging journey of caring for him and whilst I recall Elizabeth talking about Norman and the issues she was having; in truth, until I read the first draft of this book, I did not realise quite how desperate Norman's situation was and the appalling stress Elizabeth was suffering trying to manage decent care for him.

Those of us who have personally shared at least part of Elizabeth and Norman's trials recognise the truth in her multiple assertions that the information and services are out there, but visibility and access is subject to too much individual research and a dogged refusal to give in when barriers are erected.

During our first meeting I realised there were several issues that weren't right: the conflict of interest with Norman's existing investment adviser acting as an attorney; the lack of control Elizabeth was able to exercise on Norman's care without a Health and Welfare Lasting Power of Attorney; and, most importantly, her need for even more specialist advice than I could offer, to challenge the obvious failure of the NHS to pick up the ongoing cost of Norman's health (not social) care.

To address the latter, I introduced Elizabeth to Bernie Crean of Care Review Services Ltd and Angela Sherman's outstanding website 'Care to be Different'.

These three challenges to Norman receiving 'best care' were unnecessary and, had existing guidelines and best practice been followed, all avoidable. The lack of so many organisations adherence to putting the needs of not only the patient/client but also the relatives responsible for the actual 'quality of life' support first, is more than disappointing.

Norman's story is a very poignant and a sad indictment on the impact of the conflict between the NHS and local authorities in trying to avoid accepting responsibility for care. It illustrates that it takes more than just dedicated individuals and needs the support and structure of all the linked health and care organisations working in synergy to get good patient outcomes. Unfortunately, the examples of such joined-up thinking across the NHS and the health and care peripheries were severely lacking for Norman.

Elizabeth's experience of the limitations inherent in trying to get the best care outcomes for Norman without the requisite Health & Welfare LPA, compounded by the questionable appointment of a trustee with a conflict of interest in the Property & Financial LPA, could and should have been avoided. In my opinion Norman's story should be mandatory reading for all legal and financial professionals, to ensure they understand the value of the right documentation and consequences of wrong or non-existent attorney papers. My experience is, regretfully, that far too often practitioners in these two groups fail to adequately explain or push hard enough to get both LPA's arranged. In reality, for most people who need the protection, they become more important than the Will, which is so often the default focus.

I am pleased that in some small way HarperLees contributed to Elizabeth's quest for getting Norman's unsound decision of non-eligibility for NHS Continuing Healthcare overturned.

The experience and knowledge I have gained from the following three areas of my life:-

- being a Later Life Accredited Advisor (SOLLA)
- a Chartered Financial Planner

- and probably the most influential - having cared for members of my own family

all highlight and demonstrate to me just how relevant Elizabeth's book is to all parties acting in the various sectors (financial : legal : medical : care). Also, having read the book myself I found it to be an emotional and moving story. For these reasons, I will do everything in my power using my expertise as a specialist and my contacts within SOLLA to promote Elizabeth's book to the relevant sectors and the general public. Our goal – to raise the awareness of ensuring the correct legal documentation and specialist advice is in place before the worst happens.

I hope this book achieves the exposure it deserves and helps other people avoid the incredible experience suffered by Norman.

Adrian Quick Later Life Accredited Adviser (SOLLA) Chartered Financial Planner HarperLees

Preface

Whilst visiting Norman one day at the neurological nursing home, I met a very warm and understanding man called Malcolm who asked me about Norman and he listened intently to our story. During our conversation he expressed a great deal of sympathy and, at one point, he added, glibly, "You should write a book". I laughed and said "Why?" and thought little more of it.

However, as time passed, I began to realise that every one of the sectors now involved in Norman's care (medical, nursing home, home care, financial, legal) believed that they were 100% responsible for Norman and only their opinions and views counted. It appeared that, as far as they were concerned, I had no power or say regarding Norman's psychological wellbeing, quality of life, or care. As a sister, and his next of kin, my only responsibility to Norman was merely to visit him periodically and to supply whatever provisions were asked of me. Throughout the journey, knowing that Norman wanted me to care for him and that he had made people aware of this fact, I could not understand why everyone I met in the process constantly raised obstacles and hurdles for me to overcome in my quest to fulfill my promise to Norman to get him home to live with us.

Soon, from my point of view, every conversation or meeting regarding Norman's welfare bordered confrontational and compromised whether or not I would be able to keep my promise to him. I kept asking myself "Why is this process so difficult, challenging, prolonged and stressful?" More and more, Malcolm's comment began to haunt me "You should write a book", and questions started to niggle and fester in my mind "Could I, should I, try to raise awareness of the numerous issues I found myself confronted with throughout this journey?" "Could I possibly lessen the stress for somebody else finding themselves in a similar situation?" I decided to try and "Who Can Care For Me Now?" was born.

Acknowledgements

My first acknowledgement must go to my husband who was steadfastly by my side from the day I found Norman collapsed. They shared many hours together fishing, fixing cars, and the odd drink or two down the pub. To him, Norman's passing was the loss of a good and reliable friend as well as a brother-in-law and, like me, he felt that Norman did not deserve to suffer in the way that he did. Many have said how lucky I am that my husband was so "patient and understanding" but few actually realise that he was instrumental in bringing Norman home. It only took him one visit to Norman in the neurological nursing home, to recognise how unhappy Norman was and he could not bear the thought of Norman spending the rest of his life in there. Witnessing the many difficulties in achieving Norman's home-coming and care, he too was supportive of writing "Who Can Care For Me Now?" and provided me with many very welcome cups of tea, meals and the odd glass of wine! He never complained regarding the amount of time I sat at my computer writing. As always the phrase "Thank you" is an insufficient expression for the support and encouragement he has given. I know, however, that his reward was seeing Norman at home and he has no regrets regarding Norman being with us.

It would be wrong of me not to offer my thanks and appreciation to Malcolm Walker for his inspiration to write the book. He enthusiastically offered to be one of my initial guinea pigs in reading the first drafts and offered encouragement to publish. I haven't come up with a better phrase so – "Thank you Malcolm."

I would like to acknowledge the professional help, advice, and support, afforded to me by Adrian Quick of HarperLees who confirmed my belief that I was not paranoid regarding my fraught relationship with Norman's Financial Advisor, who had been appointed Joint Financial Attorney for Norman's financial affairs by his Investment Bank's solicitors. Adrian reassured me that my feelings were justified.

Adrian also took on board the challenging position I was in regarding Norman's care and pointed me in the direction of Bernie Crean of Care Review Services Ltd. Bernie, in turn, put me in touch with Stephanie Ford of Care Necessities Ltd who listened patiently and diligently to my pleas of needing more information regarding NHS Continuing Healthcare. Both Bernie and Stephanie together with an extraordinary website "Care to be Different" were instrumental in my achieving to overturn the unsound decision made by our local NHS Continuing Healthcare Team who found Norman not eligible for Continuing Healthcare. Norman's case was not even border line, he was well within the limits of eligibility but it still took a four-year battle to finally overturn their decision. In February 2018, the Independent Review Panel found Norman 100% eligible from March 2014 the day we discharged him from the neurological nursing home.

Last, but not least, Adrian has also extended great understanding and support for the relevance of writing and publishing "Who Can Care For Me Now?" Two words mean a great deal – "Thank you" to Adrian Quick, Bernie Crean, Stephanie Ford and "Care to be Different".

PART ONE
Our Story

Chapter 1
My Big Brov

Big Norm, the gentle giant, is how many of his friends described him. To me, he was my "Big Brov" nicknamed "Norm-me-man". A tall 6'3" broad chap, at his heaviest weighing 19 stone, not at all athletic but very strong – in fact, just an ordinary chap with his faults like us all, very slightly on the self-centred side having never married but soft-hearted, caring for all wildlife and never confrontational. To Mum and Dad he was their first born, Norman. Our mother came from Motherwell, just outside Glasgow and our father was a "true-blue" cockney. What a mixture we both were Glaswegian and Cockney, but it proved a wonderful mix for us both. We enjoyed a happy childhood and one of my early memories is being the pesky baby sister annoying Norman when his friend Ant (who became Norman's fishing partner and oldest friend) visited and wanted to play cards. Norman was far more intelligent than I and had attended high school and acquired several high qualifications, whilst I went to secondary modern and followed my mother's wish to become a secretary.

As the years went by we developed our own lives. I married at 19, while Norman never married and stayed at home with Mum and Dad, enjoying a bachelor life and indulging in many hobbies such as photography, fishing, bird watching, World War II aeroplanes and much more. Apart from studying accountancy after I married, my hobby became owning a horse and competing at dressage. Although brother and sister, we lived our own separate lives, each enjoying our very different hobbies, only really seeing each other at Christmas, but we did possess an underlying understanding (although never voiced) that if either of us needed help, the other would drop everything and come running.

Dad died in 1984 and Norman took this very badly but, still living at home, he was a great strength and comfort to Mum as she did not have to learn to live alone. In 1987, much to our Mum's annoyance, Norman resigned from his position as Chief Designer with a reasonably large firm and started his own business with Terence, who also resigned from his position with the same Company as Sales Director. It was agreed that Terence would look after the sales of the Company; Norman would be the person designing test equipment to measure the amperage of electricity, and Terence's partner would carry out the administration tasks. When I first met Terence it struck me how different Terence and Norman were. Norman the conventional short-back-and-sides guy, very well spoken due to his high-school education, whilst Terence appearing more trendy and in touch with the era with his long hair and hippy-style dress. To me they were chalk and cheese but they had formed a friendship which evolved into a great and successful business partnership.

Terence told me one day how annoyed and irritated he often became with Norman when new equipment arrived. Terence would spend time trying to get it to work whilst Norman appeared to be just sitting, reading. Terence said that at some point (usually when his patience was exhausted) Norman would come over and set up the equipment first time, within a few minutes. It frustrated Terence no end – Norman had been reading (once) and absorbing the instruction manual; but this was Norman extremely intellectual and a "bookworm". If his nose wasn't in an educational magazine then he was watching an educational programme, he never spent any time frivolously which is, for me, what made his last 29 months of life, suffering from a brain disease, so wicked, mother nature is so incredibly cruel.

After a few sticky years, the business flourished and became a great success. In fact it is still trading today. In approximately 2003, Norman approached Terence and said that he no longer wanted to carry out the difficult tasks within the company but would be willing to do the easier tasks. Within a short time, Norman was saying that he could not cope with the easy tasks anymore and wanted to retire completely, leaving Terence feeling very shocked and bemused, but they agreed and Norman left the company knowing that, providing he was careful, he had sufficient funds to last him throughout retirement. With the benefit of hindsight I think this was the start of Norman's dreadful brain disease as he was gradually losing motivation, focus and concentration. Our mother was, by now, suffering from a heart condition and Norman, still living at home, took most of the burden of looking after her. Mum died 2005 leaving Norman to fend for himself at home and, by now, he had been diagnosed with rheumatoid arthritis and shortly afterwards type II diabetes. I still recall and laugh at when the doctor had asked Norman if rheumatoid arthritis was in his family and Norman replied "Well it is now!" – that was Norman's sense of humour. I lived within walking distance and as soon as Mum died I suggested Norman come to us every Thursday for a meal and obviously spend Christmas with us which he readily accepted. The only time he did not come is when he went to a committee meeting of the Bomber Group in Suffolk – another serious hobby of his.

Over the next years, we did not see much of a decline in Norman until 2012 but we had commented that he no longer went out and about and when I said to him "Hi brov, what have you been up to this week?" he replied "Nothing". Come October 2012 when coming round to ours we noticed a serious decline in his mobility. He was now finding it very difficult to walk, stand up and sit down. Also he was losing feeling and movement in his left hand. I found out later that both Terence and Ant were nagging Norman to go to the doctors and so was I as he could no longer open a packet of crisps himself or cut his own food up.

It was now Christmas Day 2012 about 12.30 p.m., dinner was cooking and we were waiting for Norman to arrive. His mobility had been deteriorating recently but he had said he would walk round. The doorbell rang and I went to answer it. There was Norman, his face drawn, his breathing shallow, holding on to the top of the front door. Although he had lost a lot of weight he was still 6'3" and filled the doorway. He stumbled in the door and steadied himself by reaching up to the ceiling. Kevin (my husband) came running and we managed to get Norman into the living room and sit him on a dining room chair. Kevin and I were both shocked at how distressed Norman was but he seemed to improve once sitting.

Christmas dinner was about ready, so we cut it up for Norman as we knew he had difficulty in using his left hand and we all sat around the table eating. Norman polished off his Christmas meal – appetite did not appear to be a problem at this stage. We cleared the table and sat on the sofas to watch the same old Christmas TV but Norman remained on the chair. He struggled a few times but could not get up which was new to us. We asked if he wanted us to help and he said "Yes". So we helped him to his feet and he shuffled across to a recliner chair and made himself comfy.

Worried, I now started to nag and said that things had gone far enough. I was making an appointment with the doctor this week and he was going. Norman argued saying that the doctor(s) had made no difference and he had an appointment with a specialist middle to late January for his rheumatoid arthritis, which we all thought must be the reason for the decline in his mobility. I said he was going!

First thing Boxing Day, we took an electric "riser" chair which was sitting unused in the garage around to Norman which we believed would help him get to his feet. We were surprised, however, when we witnessed Norman having difficulty using the buttons. Not only did it seem difficult physically for him to use the buttons, but mentally he did not appear to grasp what to do and we had to keep reminding him. This was not the Norman I knew and concerned me greatly but I, simply, did not understand why it was so difficult for him.

I had not visited Mum and Dad's bungalow for some time (and to this day, I feel guilty about this) as Norman now always came to us and I was shocked at how untidy it was. I spent most of Christmas week cleaning and moaning (I'm good at that – well practiced!) at Norman, saying that he could not live like this – he needed help.

I telephoned the doctors and the receptionist who answered informed me that the doctor would not see Norman upon my request. Being a patient myself I made an appointment for myself and took Norman with me. Once the doctor realised how worried I was regarding Norman he was more than happy to see both of us together. He was very sympathetic and saw for himself how stiff and immobile Norman had become. The doctor, like us, was fixated on Norman's rheumatoid arthritis and said he would give Norman an injection to help him get to the specialist's appointment. Norman forcibly said "The injections make no difference." The doctor said he would give him a double injection of steroids. Injection given, there was little improvement. For the next couple of weeks I went round to Norman's every day, prepared him something to eat and did some cleaning (not my forte!).

Norman continued to move around the bungalow on his own two feet, albeit slow and awkward. I asked about him falling as I was worried but he replied that he never felt like he was about to fall. Tuesday, 22nd January 2013, my car was in for service and I was at work. I rang Norman – no answer. This was not unusual but made me uneasy. I finished work at 5 p.m. and drove straight round to Norman's. Instantly, I knew something was wrong. The bedroom and bathroom lights were on, the milk was still on the doorstep and the post in the letter box. We had been brought up with the front door always left unlocked and as I entered, I found Norman crumpled in a heap almost in a sitting position on the bathroom floor. I gasped "How long have you been like that?", he said it had happened during the night. I said to him he had no choice, I was ringing for an ambulance and he was going into hospital and hopefully they will sort him out.

Chapter 2
Hospital

The ambulance was dispatched (not on blues) and I chatted to Norman awaiting its arrival. Whilst waiting, I asked him if he had eaten the food I had left him in the fridge. He replied that I had not left him anything. I looked in the fridge and there it was untouched and I remember thinking to myself "Why has Norman forgotten?" I asked him and Norman replied that I had not told him. The ambulance arrived within an hour or so and a female and a male paramedic came to help. The bathroom was small which made picking Norman up off the floor difficult. He had soiled himself and was now sick bringing up urine as his kidneys were failing. The female paramedic kept finding excuses not to move Norman as she couldn't cope with urine and faeces but she was OK with blood. The paramedics also stated that they did not have the correct equipment on board to lift Norman and toyed with the idea of calling another ambulance but didn't. Eventually, about an hour and half later the male paramedic showed his frustration at the female paramedic and said "Look we have got to get this chap to hospital." They manoeuvred him and eventually moved him into the ambulance. It was a further 20 minutes or more before they moved off. I think they were trying to get a line into him. I waited until they left, locked the bungalow, picked Kevin up and we drove to the hospital. We arrived at the hospital and as we were walking down the corridor a doctor shouted from behind "Get out of my way." Later I learnt he was rushing to Norman. On arrival at the hospital, Norman suffered a blood pressure arrest; he was toxic with the diabetes and rheumatoid arthritis drugs he had taken with insufficient food. His kidneys failed completely, he was hypothermic and dehydrated and possibly had an infection. A doctor came and spoke to us and said the next couple of hours were critical.

Feeling shocked and numb, we waited in the waiting room until the early hours of the next day when another doctor came in and invited us to accompany Norman to intensive care and we stayed with him for a while.

Intensive Care

After what seems a couple of sleepless hours, it is the next day and I am on my way to see Norman in intensive care. There is very little restriction on visiting hours so you can go when you like. Driving to the hospital I am left with my thoughts, wondering what I am about to walk into. The question "How did we get here?" spinning round and round my head like a broken record. Once outside intensive care you ring to be allowed in. It seemed an eternity but finally I am asked who I am, and who am I visiting, and allowed in. There is Norman, still and silent, lying in his bed. Tubes everywhere but it is so reassuring when you realise his care is one-to-one. I talked to the nurse who said he had had a good night. She constantly kept him comfy, using extraction to clear his throat. He is so still showing no signs of restlessness or movement at all. We have never been a touchy-feely family and I find it difficult now, but I take his hand his eyes open, and I comfort him the best I can. It's difficult to know what to do or what to say, but I sit close to him and talk to the nurse. At least he knows I am there and can listen to my voice.

It is amazing how quickly seriously-ill people can rally round in intensive care. Within 48 hours, Norman starts to look better. I visit him every day feeling that although there is very little I can do, it must be horrid to be in hospital with no visitors and feeling alone. After ten days – which I was told is a long stay in intensive care as people usually only stay four to five days – I am informed that Norman is to be moved to a ward. I felt relieved. At least now he is out of danger. How wrong I was!

The Ward

I am driving to the hospital again taking some comfort that Norman is now in a ward and not in intensive care. I walk down the corridors constantly wondering what I was going to find. Once in the ward I am looking for Norman. He looks better and acknowledges me. There is a tray in front of him with his meal on it. He cannot reach it or cut it up and so, naturally, I help him to eat his meal. He is in a side ward on his own with next to no company. He can talk to me but cannot turn himself on to his side, or sit up. He can move his legs and arms slightly but cannot weight bear. I continue to visit every day and he continues to improve slightly. I manage to talk to a doctor regarding his lack of movement and asked regarding his diagnosis and prognosis. "Will he get his movement back? What quality of life will he have?". The doctor asks for the history and I give him as much information as I can. He tells me that unless they are able to reverse what has happened to Norman, his quality of life will be what I see. I'm shell shocked and have great difficulty in processing this information. My head had always been in the sand and I did not understand what can happen to a person who has been taken so seriously ill. The doctor explains that the breakdown of Norman's muscles has been "off the scale" and they are still continuing to break down. Within the next couple of days I visit Norman and my hopes are raised as when I walk into him, he exclaims "I've been standing up today." He is so happy. The physiotherapist had been in and placed Norman on a board so although he had been upright, he had been fully supported. We chatted that night more than usual as his hopes had been raised.

The next day as I drive to the hospital, I feel slightly happier remembering Norman the night before. As I walk into the side ward, the sister of the ward was feeding Norman. He looked semi-conscious, white and very drawn. I asked what was going on and she replied that Norman was having difficulty feeding himself and so she was helping. I asked what had happened. She said "Nothing." I said "He had been standing up on a board the day before and the change in him is significant, so something must have happened". She said she did not know as she had not been working the day before and had not seen him. I said "Well I saw him the day before and the change is too significant. Has he seen a doctor?". She said "No". I said "He must see a doctor to make sure he is not suffering from a stroke or something". She appeared not to want to call a doctor as it was now around 6 p.m. and doctors finish at 5 p.m., but I insisted. She said she would put a call out. A while later she came back and said that a doctor would come but it will be a couple of hours and suggested I went home. She said she did not finish her shift until 9 p.m. and would give me a ring. Norman appeared not to know whether or not I was there and so I decided to drive home. My mind is working overtime whilst driving home as I am thinking that; had Norman been at home, I could have rung 999 or parcelled him into a car and taken him to A&E. I waited until 8.30 p.m. – no phone call. I called the ward and spoke to the sister. She confirmed that no doctor had been. I reiterated my concern explaining how worried I was and insisted again that he see a doctor. She said she would call a doctor and ring me back. I couldn't believe that Norman was in hospital and could not see a doctor. Where is the logic? She rang back 9.15 pm and confirmed that Norman had seen a doctor and he was fine. I had another sleepless night. I knew Norman was not "fine".

On my way to hospital the next day, obviously I was re-living the night before. As I enter Norman's side-room I was met by his consultant. Norman was worse. They were going to transfer him to the "high-dependency" ward. I asked what was wrong. Little information was given and I accompanied Norman to the "high-dependency" ward. Immediately I felt better as I realised that the care ratio is two-to-three patients to one nurse. The next day during my visit, I am trying to glean some information as to what has gone wrong – how can someone's condition change so rapidly and nobody notice until the patient needs to be transferred to "high-dependency"? Finally, I am told that Norman has suffered an internal bleed and is being given a blood transfusion. He stayed in the "high-dependency" ward for approximately five days and received eight units of blood. Norman was then transferred back to the ward – to a ratio of 12 or more patients to one nurse.

I continued to visit Norman everyday as the routine seemed to be that his food would be left on a tray out of reach. In himself he seemed to be improving slightly. After a couple of weeks his kidneys had recovered and were working well but he still could hardly move. I tried to talk to the consultant of the ward but struggled. Eventually he spoke to me and I asked what was going on. The ward Norman was on was for kidney failure. His kidneys were now working fine. It appeared his problem now may be neurological. The days passed by one by one. I visited Norman; he made me laugh by moaning about the old lady in the cubicle next door shouting continuously "Help." He was impatient of her making a fuss and thought she should "shut up". Within a day or two, it became the routine that the nurses relied upon me to turn up every day to help Norman eat which, at least, gave me something to do whilst there. Like all relatives I went in with "goodies" – flavoured water, magazines, food, clothing, etc., and I "clocked" that Norman did not look at any of his magazines which was not like the Norman I knew. A month passed by, Norman's back was itching every night and he kept asking me to scratch the itches which was fine but I was worried I would scratch his skin off.

Norman has been in hospital now for between four to six weeks, and I was beginning to find it time consuming and irritating to ensure that I had £21 in £1 coins every week to pay the car parking fees of £3 per day. I went to PALS (Patient Advice and Liaison Service) and they informed me that parking was free for long-staying patients and issued me with a one-week pass. By now I'm struggling at work with the amount of time I'm taking off and can only visit after work hours. The weekly ticket, however, can only be reissued during work hours. On discussing my dilemma with PALS, they put me in touch with the Manager of the car park facilities who, I have to say, is probably the person with the most common sense I have met throughout this whole process. He issued monthly tickets by email. What continues to frustrate me though is that this facility like so many others is not adequately advertised – you have to find out for yourself!

It is now approximately six weeks and Norman is still in the ward. The daily routine is firmly established. Nothing is happening. I try my hardest to talk to the consultant; he will not talk to me as his expertise is "kidneys". His secretary refers me to the neurologist. I try to contact the neurologist whose secretary told me that he only carries out clinics at the hospital and referred me back to the consultant. Finally, its back to PALS delivering a complaint letter.

As a result of talking to PALS, the neurologist agreed to talk to me and made an appointment for me at his day clinic. He explained that Norman's consultant had asked him to visit Norman, as the hospital did not employ a neurologist (so why wasn't Norman transferred to a hospital who had a neurologist?). He asked me to give him as much history as possible and I left after approximately half an hour having gleaned little information apart from the fact that it was probably the double-steroid injection which was the last straw for Norman's body and caused his collapse. The neurologist also informed me that the hospital is going to carry out a muscle biopsy.

I continue to visit Norman and, in himself, he is not too bad. It is now several weeks, and I feel for Norman as he has not seen any television, and only listened to a little radio. Surely, he must need some form of entertainment and/or stimuli. There is no point in me putting money into the television as Norman cannot switch it on or off, change stations or move it (it is often left out of reach). Naturally, I turn the radio on for him when I visit but the next time I visit it is not only turned off, but often placed well out of reach. I ask the nursing staff if they could turn the radio on for him and they replied "OK" but it never happened. I take a Walkman in and some cassettes with speaking books but Norman will not/can not work this for himself and so I decide to play one for him whilst visiting in the afternoon. This highlights that he finds difficulty in concentrating for any length of time and fatigues very quickly and so I look for an alternative. I encourage his friends to visit, especially Terence and Ant, as this really gives Norman a lift, but they find it difficult to see him like this. Norman, missing his friends, said to me one night "Tell them I'm dead. They will come to my funeral", and grinned.

During my visits, he is still continuously "itching" and wants me to scratch the itches and I'm worried about taking his skin off but do the best I can by rubbing his back with his bed robe and he reminds me of a bear scratching his back on a tree. On mentioning this abnormal itching to the medical staff, I receive no response or help. I help him brush his teeth and eat his meals. His kidneys are now working well, but the hospital continue to be concerned regarding muscle wastage. The result of the muscle biopsy is normal and I try to talk to the consultant, neurologist, doctor – anyone – but no one will speak to me. I approach PALS yet again and ask for some information regarding Norman. Eventually, a consultant agrees to talk to me and tells me that it will take months for Norman's muscles to recover, physiotherapy is not working and so they are no longer giving him any.

It is now early March 2013 and there is talk of discharging Norman. He will have to go into a care home because his many conditions include him being fully immobile and double incontinent, requiring a large bedroom downstairs to house a hospital bed, ceiling hoist and wet room, plus the property must be fully accessible inside and outside to a large, heavy, wheelchair. Unfortunately, it is impossible to care for him in either of our homes as both were too small to carry out the necessary adaptations. On discussing this with Norman, clearly he was anxious and scared and who could blame him?

One evening when we were discussing it he said to me "I want to be one of your horses", a comment which really hit home, as I knew exactly what he was trying to say but I had no idea how this comment would resonate with me from this day forward.

For years, Norman had witnessed my compassion for life. For me life is not a rehearsal. It is fragile and can be distinguished all too easily and should be cherished. He had seen for himself no expense spared whether it be money or time and effort to maximise my horses' quality of life, especially towards the end of their life. He had witnessed my tears when I had stayed with one particular horse throughout the night, as he called to me the second I left his stable, until the vet came the next day and, the last thing I could do for the horse was to hold his head collar and stay with him, whilst the vet put him to sleep. Norman had also seen how I looked after another horse which developed a condition very similar to diabetes. With the benefit of hindsight, I think this is the one-to-one, quality care, empathy, understanding, and compassion, Norman was hoping to receive himself. He did not want to be left alone in a hospital bed or care home, feeling deserted and abandoned.

Initially, having no idea what the future held, I reacted jovially saying "So you want to live in a stable? Well, you know we have one spare." But now I wonder if he had had a better idea than me as to what the future did hold. Did he know that his care would leave a lot to be desired? Had he witnessed this for himself whilst visiting friends in hospital and care homes as he so often had? Naively, at that time, I had no reason to question the care world (ignorance is bliss), but clearly he felt that my horses had better care than he was experiencing or expecting to receive from a care home and sadly time and events proved him to be right.

Today, having shared Norman's journey from collapse to death and witnessing for myself all types of care available (hospital, nursing home, live-in, pop-in and private) whenever I remember Norman's request to be one of my horses it provokes so many questions I can not answer relating to the services provided by the medical and care sectors of our society.

During one of my visits, I am asked to contact the discharge team which I manage to do quite quickly. I cannot believe it; within the first ten words with her she says "If there is a house – it will have to be sold to pay for his care." I was so angry, I replied, "And what happens if he makes a miraculous recovery?" I could not believe the callousness of her attitude. How dare they tell me or Norman what to do financially!

I made an appointment to visit the nearest care home and looked around their facilities. It is difficult to put into words what I saw but I decided that I did not want Norman to go there. Within a few months this particular care home featured on the news programme *Panorama* reporting on inadequate care and ill treatment of patients and I was so pleased I had disregarded it. I talked this over further with Norman and he said that he knew the owner of another local care home and to visit that one. I never arranged to visit the second care home because, sadly, events over took us.

Intensive Care Two

The hospital decided that before discharging Norman, he should visit a specialist hospital in Cambridge for further investigations into his lack of mobility, and made an appointment for him for approximately three weeks' time. Leading up to the appointment date I continued the daily routine of visiting, helping Norman eat, brush his teeth, etc. One week away from his appointment, the specialist hospital postponed it until the second week in April. The Thursday before Easter weekend, I visited Norman as per normal to find him not himself. He was very uncomfortable around his private parts. I approached the nurse on duty and was greeted with the indifference I had come to expect. Clearly, Norman was uncomfortable and I was extremely concerned. Norman seemed to want to try to rest and he told me that I might as well go home which again was very unusual as he normally liked the company even if we did not talk too much. I approached the nurse again and she assured me she would look at him. There was no point in me asking for a doctor as I had been there a few weeks back and I knew what their response would be.

During the drive home I was so worried, it seemed a complete repeat of what had happened a few weeks earlier when he had suffered an internal bleed which had been ignored until he needed to be transferred to the high-dependency ward. On arrival at home, I said to Kevin, "Norman really isn't well and I'm expecting a telephone call". The telephone call came about 4 p.m. the next day (Good Friday). An urgent call, informing me that Norman is extremely poorly and to make my way to the hospital as a matter of urgency. When I arrived 30 minutes later, Norman was clearly distressed with the "crash" team of approximately 20 people surrounding him. He was on oxygen and his breathing seemed poor. Despite all of the people and equipment surrounding him I could see his eyes looking at me asking for reassurance – I could do nothing but stand by and watch. The whole atmosphere was surreal, like an episode from a soap television programme. After what seemed an eternity, the decision was made to move Norman to intensive care. The handover was made and we were sent to get a coffee and then ushered to the relations' waiting room. Eventually, a consultant came to talk to us and said that this was the third time Norman had been transferred to an intensive/high-dependency ward and it was Norman's last time – three strikes and out! I could not believe what I was hearing and struggled to come to terms with the implications. The consultant went away and said he would return. Upon his return he said that Norman had septicaemia and would probably bounce back fairly quickly, certainly in time to keep his appointment at the specialist hospital. We were taken to see Norman and the consultant told me to hold his hand and talk to him. Norman looked petrified and who could blame him? My heart went out to him. I asked him to squeeze my hand if he could understand me and I felt a soft squeeze. I told him that he had septicaemia and he would get better. I also told him that I would do everything in my power to ensure that he would come home to live with us. He squeezed my hand softly. Bizarrely, despite Norman being in a critical ward, I went home being slightly comforted because I knew he was being looked after to the best of anyone's ability and not just left alone in a side ward being visited and checked upon who knows when.

Norman's stay in intensive care was only for a few days and one evening when I pushed the bell outside intensive care to be allowed in, the head nurse said she would be out to talk to me. She informed me that Norman had been transferred back to the ward where he had come from which was a renal ward (his kidneys by now were working fine) and, clearly, he was in the wrong ward for his current condition. My legs went to jelly, I was hot and cold and felt sick. Tears started to flow uncontrollably down my cheeks as I exclaimed "Oh no, please not there they will kill him!" Aghast and shocked at my outburst; immediately, the nurse ushered me out of the corridor and away from other relations waiting to go in, through the intensive care ward and into a side room. She asked me to explain and I told her of our experiences in the ward including not recognising his internal bleed until 24 hours later than myself and also not noticing this episode. She went away and came back with a consultant and asked me to explain all over again. I was given a cup of tea and the usual words of comfort when someone is so distressed. They said that I must go to PALS and that they would take it up further themselves.

Back To The Ward

Slightly calmer, I made my way to the ward and was shocked to see Norman. He was so, so, so, poorly, shouting "Help me"; "Help me." I went to the nurses' station and was told that he had had a stroke. He was extremely thirsty but not allowed to drink. He kept shouting at me "Why won't you help me? Help me." A young doctor came in and it seemed to me that he too was very stressed at the whole scenario and stayed with us for a while. He apologised saying that there was only one nurse on duty and twelve side wards let alone the main ward. I could not believe that Norman was transferred from the intensive care ward in such a state. It kept going through my mind; there was Norman in intensive care with one-to-one nursing and then, literally, within five minutes he was on a ward with next to no care. The young doctor said that his shift had ended some time ago, apologised and said he had to leave me alone with Norman. He genuinely seemed upset at the situation. The only thing I could do for Norman was to moisten his lips with cotton wool lollipops and just to keep trying to explain to him that I couldn't do more and hope that he took some comfort from me being there. The feeling of helplessness was unbearable. I stayed with Norman for as long as I possibly could because he was so distressed but late that night I was asked to go home. I did not like leaving Norman one little bit.

After being asked to leave, I left the hospital to drive home. My mind going over and over what had happened tonight. I just could not understand why a person so ill and so distressed would be moved from such a closely-monitored situation of one-to-one care in ITU (Intensive Therapy Unit) to the exact opposite in a side ward, with a staff ratio of one nurse to at least 12 patients and no doctor. I kept remembering what I had said to Norman when I found him collapsed, "Well at least I can get you into hospital now where you will be looked after" – what a joke, how wrong could I have been? People say over and over "Hospital is the best place" – well it wasn't for Norman! This night I realised so many things. The high majority of hospital staff are caring people who want to do a good job but they are so hindered by the system and lack of staff.

It also seemed very strange to me that hospital staff went out of their way to encourage visitors to complain to PALS. I appeared to live at the PALS office complying with the requests from staff to complain. After a couple of visits, the PALS staff explained, defensively, that they had little power to actually help. Their remit was to communicate complaints to the correct department which they assured me they would do and then it was down to the department to react. A few days later, PALS informed me that they had been able to arrange a meeting between myself, two doctors from Norman's ward, the sister of the ward, and a secretary who would take notes. I took an afternoon off work as holiday and went along to the meeting, well prepared with a long list of my concerns, some statistics regarding patient ratio numbers, and I also wanted to express my own feelings that "tick lists" had replaced individual's responsibility and the old-fashioned nursing of observation. It was now mid-April 2013 and Norman had been in hospital since January 2013. I had visited him every day without fail and felt that I was well informed regarding his care and daily routine. Some of my issues were fairly minor, (pillows placed in such a way as to force Norman's head forward, call button out of reach, food and drink left out of reach, no radio turned on); but others I felt were much more serious. I explained that this was the second time that I had noticed a serious decline in Norman's health and, despite my reporting it to the ward staff, the hospital had not reacted to the decline until Norman needed to be transferred to an intensive care ward. It was obvious from their replies that I was not fighting those present in the meeting but the NHS system(s) and perhaps this explained the ward staff's appetite for complaints to be reported to PALS. These people were working with only one doctor covering the whole of the hospital after 5 p.m during the week and one doctor throughout the whole weekend. Nursing ratios being one nurse to at least 12 patients. No continuity in staffing. Every day someone different was nursing the patient which took away responsibility. Old-fashioned nursing of observation had been replaced with "tick lists". Completion of paperwork had become more important than nursing. I mentioned to the doctors present that the ITU consultant had told me that the septicaemia had been caused by the catheter and a way round this was to use convenes as I was very concerned that Norman may get septicaemia again and I had also been told that the septicaemia had caused Norman to suffer a stroke. One of the doctors present said that it is very unlikely that Norman would get septicaemia again and I asked why. I cannot tell you how shocked and horrified I was at his reply. He told me, casually, that Norman had developed septicaemia as the result of a short-term catheter being inserted on admission on 22nd January which had not been checked or changed until Norman fell ill with septicaemia and, coupled to this, when they did change the catheter no antibiotics were given as a precaution. I also found out later that there were no records that the catheter had been inserted. So, in fact, from my point of view the hospital had saved Norman's life only to take it away from him again. Norman never "bounced back" from this episode of septicaemia and I still wonder today what difference it would have made to his quality of life had he not contracted septicaemia from the catheter being left in too long.

I was left trying to come to terms with the fact that the ITU consultant had told me that Norman had had three visits in a short space of time to ITU and would not have a fourth – only one visit was caused by actual illness – the other two had been caused by the hospital!!!

It was clear from the meeting that I was hitting my head against a brick wall because those present were not in a position to help. The sister clearly felt unjustly criticised but also had some sympathy for the position Norman and I were in. I reassured her that I thought it was the NHS system(s) that was at fault and not the staff and I urged her to push my complaint to the next level. She said that the Medical Director of the hospital would be willing to meet me if I wanted him to and she seemed very surprised by my answer "Yes I would – as soon as possible, please."

A meeting with him was arranged and I informed him of what had happened to date. He came across as a very personable person listening to what I had to say. He asked what I wanted and I said that I wanted Norman moved somewhere where he would be cared for properly and receive the correct physio. During our conversation, mention was made of the septicaemia. I asked the Medical Director if he knew what had caused it and he replied that he had not been able to read Norman's notes. I informed him of what I had been told that the septicaemia had been caused by the catheter which had not been changed from January to April. He appeared taken aback and shocked. His body language changed and became that of a very uncomfortable person recognising the implications (possible hospital negligence). I said to him that at this moment in time my only concern was for Norman's welfare and I wanted Norman to be placed in the care of a responsible doctor. The Medical Director's body language to me was clear that he wanted to end this meeting but needed to know what I wanted for Norman. I reiterated that I wanted Norman placed somewhere where he would be cared for and somewhere where someone would take responsibility for his treatment and wellbeing and somewhere where he would be given physio. I did not realise that I was actually asking the impossible! This lesson I learnt later in our journey. The Medical Director said that he could transfer Norman to the Stroke Ward as Norman had had a stroke (as a result of the septicaemia). The Medical Director said that he had a great deal of respect for the consultant on that ward and that he was an excellent doctor. Naturally, I agreed as I just wanted good care for Norman and someone to take responsibility for his treatment and recovery. The Medical Director said that he would talk to the consultant to make sure that he was willing to take Norman on as a case and that on the assumption he did, arrangements would be made for Norman to be transferred to the Stroke Ward immediately upon Norman's return from the specialist hospital. The Medical Director gave me his email address and said that I could contact him any time and then excused himself as he wanted to go and follow up on the cause of Norman's septicaemia. The Medical Director also commented during our conversation that the hospital should not be offering nursing services if it was unable to fulfil this promise. This comment endeared the Medical Director to me and reassured me that someone did care after all and, possibly, stopped me from taking further action against the hospital (a decision I now regret), as all I wanted now was for Norman to receive the quality of care that we all deserve once falling so desperately ill.

I returned to the ward to see how Norman was doing. Over the next few days he seemed to improve a little. The stroke had affected his speech, swallowing and motivation, badly. Now he was significantly worse than before the septicaemia. The intensive care consultant had said that Norman should bounce back quite quickly from the septicaemia and I just kept reminding myself of this comment and kept hoping, but it did not happen. It was expected that Norman would be well enough to keep his appointment in two weeks' time at the specialist hospital and I was told that the Medical Director would arrange for him to be moved onto the Stroke Ward upon his return. I was reassured that the consultant for the Stroke Ward would meet the criteria that I so desperately wanted for Norman being that someone would take an interest in his case and ensure that he was looked after and nursed to the best of anyone's ability (I was soon to learn that this was an empty promise!).

The next two weeks passed as before with me visiting daily to help Norman with his evening meals etc. One night, he seemed particularly low and would not feed himself so I placed the food on the fork and put the fork to his mouth and he ate it quite happily. I then heard a nurse shouting at me "What are you doing? Why are you feeding him? He can feed himself. He has managed all day until you arrived." Flabbergasted, I did not know what to say. After everything we had just been through, I was so scared that Norman would die and I did not want it on my conscience that I did not do everything I could for him. The nurse came over and asked Norman aggressively why he was insisting that I should feed him. Clearly, this verbal attack from the nurse distressed Norman (and me) and all he could say was "I don't know." I learnt later that the nurse did have a point as it is the action of hand to mouth that stimulates saliva to aid swallowing, but she was, most certainly, heartless, insensitive and clearly approached the situation in the wrong manner.

The day for the outpatients visit to the specialist hospital came and Norman was transported there. It gave me my first evening off which, I must admit, I did welcome. I was also hopeful that the specialist hospital would be able to explain what was wrong with Norman. Perhaps after his visit I would understand more and, on return, Norman would be transferred to the Stroke Ward under a consultant who had voluntarily agreed to take on his case. I felt slightly more positive.

Within hours of Norman's return and being admitted to the Stroke Ward, I visited him. I spoke to the head nurse who seemed very personable. Within two days; immediately upon my arrival at Norman's bedside I saw that he was struggling to breath, his face was a picture of sheer terror yet again. He managed to ask me what the time was and I said 6 p.m. He had asked me this as that was my normal visiting time and he was obviously thinking if I was there at any other time then he must be dying – I instantly knew the relevance of that question but obviously no one else did. A young doctor was struggling to get a line into Norman's arm and, unintentionally, I uttered out loud "This F...ing hospital." Those present were down on me like a tonne of bricks – "We don't have that language in this hospital, leave immediately." I refused and stood my ground. The head nurse came up to me, into my personal space, and tried to force me to leave. I grew roots. I was going nowhere. I tried to explain the history of the past five months in the hospital and that this was just repetition of the previous ward. No one appeared to listen, care, or even be interested. As far as they were concerned, Norman's history started two days ago and they were doing the best they could for a patient they did not know. It was a real lesson that every time Norman was moved, his history was wiped clean. My presence now made the young doctor nervous. It was far from intentional on my part but it was also useless to try to explain my emotions to anyone. I did, however, try to apologise. She failed to get a line in, which resulted in the specialist team being called to Norman's bedside. I was actually pleased, as this team got the line in in seconds and so I had, inadvertently, saved Norman a tiny amount of trauma.

As I stood there watching, three friends of Norman's arrived to visit. I had made plans with them for this visit but unfortunately events had over taken. I always feel sad that Norman never saw them as they had travelled 2½ hours to visit him and understandably they never made the trip again. When I think of this evening, I am appalled and frustrated that the only time I ever received an immediate reaction from the staff at the hospital was when I swore inadvertently – it had just slipped out under my breath as a result of my own stress, fear, and frustration, that Norman kept getting so ill from the catheter which simply was not checked/changed often enough, and it appeared that every new ward had to learn "Norman" and until they did he suffered. Norman improved within 48 hours and interestingly he was referred to urology for a bladder investigation. I was promised by the Medical Director of the hospital who agreed to transfer Norman to this (the stroke) ward that the consultant on this ward would talk to me and look after him. I made an appointment to see the consultant. I asked about the catheter, and he said that Norman's catheter would have to remain because he had stones in his bladder which would have to be removed by an operation. I mentioned that

Norman was constantly asking me to scratch his back and I did not consider this normal and the consultant said he would take care of it. I asked if Norman could see the hospital's optician as despite being a vivid reader before he fell ill, he would no longer even attempt to read any literature I brought in for him. He agreed. Despite several chases, it never happened. The routine returned to how it was in the other ward. I visited in the evening to help Norman to eat and the days passed.

I met the wife and daughter of the patient in the adjacent bed to Norman. He had been in the hospital a month or two longer than Norman, having been taken ill at Christmas with an infection that had travelled up his spine into his brain. His wife was quite distressed as he had been discharged from the hospital with "nothing wrong" only a few days before falling seriously ill. She had asked for the radio to be turned on for him and, like me, was frustrated when this did not happen.

After two weeks I asked for an appointment with the consultant. It was arranged for a week's time. I arrived a few minutes early (as you do) and went to reception to let them know I was here. I was told that no appointment had been made and the consultant was not on the ward. I made another appointment for a few days' times. I arrived a few minutes early again and was told that the consultant would see me soon. He walked up to me and acknowledged me and said he would be a few minutes. He continuously walked passed us and after one and a half hours I went up to reception to ask when he would see me. I was told he had gone home! I never had another meeting to find out how Norman was progressing or glean any knowledge regarding his various illnesses or condition.

Norman was transferred into a side room on the same ward which was a little bit of a shame really as he had made friends with the person in the adjacent bed. A couple of bed sores had broken out and so he was now regularly seen by the tissue viability nurse. I asked about physio and the optician but both requests fell on deaf ears. For me, the most frustrating part is that I am trying to do the best for my brother but nobody tells me straight – "No, you cannot see an optician or have physio", I am just left waiting, waiting, wondering, trying to work it out for myself – after all, such a large hospital has its own optician – so why? Nobody explains why they will not give physio, I am just left waiting and waiting and waiting. All I could do was push to try and get Norman out of hospital, hopefully into a better-equipped environment to cope with his many health issues. I had been told by one of the nurses that there was talk that he would be moved to a neurological nursing home. When I prompted for more information, they said they were not sure. I asked where the home was, its name, anything (after all I would be Norman's main visitor), it was like drawing blood out of a stone. Finally, someone gave me the name and I was able to look it up on the internet. It was approximately 30 miles away and one of only two NHS Neurological Nursing Homes in the country.

One morning I received a telephone call from the hospital saying that Norman had been transferred to the Burns Ward as they had had an emergency stroke patient admitted overnight. After all of my fighting to get Norman into this ward, the promises that he would be looked after by the consultant, etc.; as quick as a flash he was transferred overnight – yes, I know, if they need the bed, they need the bed. I surprised myself by actually being OK about this news. I was beginning to learn and possibly even accept that I have no say or influence on Norman's care, even when it is poor and well below standard.

That night as usual, I made my way to see Norman. When I entered the ward he was in a side ward opposite the nurses' station. The ward itself was one of the most pleasant, light, airy, roomy, and even quite cheery. As I entered and said "Hi" to Norm, very quickly it became evident that mentally he was in a bad place, something I had never witnessed before. He was angry, yet tearful, snapping at every word I said. He told me that he had been moved to the wrong ward. I went over to the nurses' desk and was told that the ward sister wanted to talk to me so I waited and waited and waited as I had come to expect. Finally she approached me and addressed me in a loud, hostile, voice, "Why has your brother been moved to this ward? We do not have the nursing skills, or the equipment for someone with his disabilities? We are a burns unit, not a stroke unit. You need to complain to PALS and ask for him to be transferred. We do not understand why he was transferred here. We cannot look after him." This was all shouted in the hearing distance of Norman. He heard every word. Now I understood why his mood was so down. It was the first time I had ever seen him so low and it was the first of many times I witnessed him crying.

I told the sister that as soon as I arrived home I would email the hospital's Medical Director and tell him what she had said. She appeared to physically take a step back and her face drained of colour. I think my response was a great deal more than she had bargained for. Two other people during my visit came up to me and snapped at me saying that I must contact PALS as this was a Burns Ward which did not have the staff, skills or equipment to cope with Norman's disabilities and, therefore, they could not look after him.

I went back in and tried to cheer Norman up. During his illness he had received many, many emails from his American friends being members of the Bomber Group based in Suffolk, as well as his many friends from his work and his hobbies such as fishing, photography, wildlife, etc. I had received notification that the owner of the bomber Sally B had arranged to include well wishes to Norman during its next flight around the airfield sites in southern Britain. They were also trying to fit in a fly-past of the hospital to say Hi to Norman in recognition of his hard work raising money to keep Sally B flying. As I started to tell him, his face crumbled and started to crack, tears welled up in his eyes and he started to sob; blurting out between sobs that they are all probably dead by now. I was frozen. I had failed to cheer him up, I had just made it worse. I looked over to him and saw the shell of the brother I had grown up with. My 6'3", 19-stone older brother was sobbing his heart out and there was *nothing* I could do. I had not witnessed this before. Nurses came in and tried to console him. Naturally, I stayed until he had quietened down and stopped crying.

Looking back, sometimes I wonder how I managed to drive home constantly filled with every emotion you can imagine. My brother had been taken so seriously ill and I did not understand why and I had not been able to gain any information from the medical staff. I can only assume they did not know either. He had been given a double steroid injection at Christmas which was the wrong thing to do and I had been the one to push Norman to go to the doctors. The ambulance paramedics had taken so long in lifting him from the bathroom floor because they kept saying they did not have the right equipment on board. It had taken them about 1½ hours! He was admitted with hypothermia, dehydration, infection, extremely low blood pressure, kidney failure and toxic poisoning from taking medicated drugs with insufficient food and drink. The hospital saved his life only to leave him in a ward where they chose to ignore me when I asked what was wrong with him when he deteriorated significantly within 24 hours. He had an internal bleed which they ignored until he needed eight units of blood and transferred him to the high-dependency ward. They transferred him back to the ward only to ignore my pleas yet again a few weeks later, when I said he was deteriorating, until he was suffering from severe septicaemia caused by inserting a catheter on admission and not recording it and therefore ignoring it, and not changing it until it caused septicaemia which then caused a stroke. I had fought and fought to get him transferred to what I thought was a more suitable ward with better care, and here I was back to square one. He was now in a ward where the actual sister of the ward and nurses all said they did not have the staff, skills or equipment, to look after him. I remembered my words to Norman the day I found him collapsed, which were "Well brov, now you have no option, I'm getting you into hospital where you will be looked after properly until you recover. After all, hospital is the best place for you." Those words continuously echoed through me – how wrong could I be?! It was a long and exhausting drive home.

As soon as I arrived home, I emailed the Medical Director of the hospital. My email was short and curt as, right or wrong, I was so, so, angry as to how any human being could be treated in this way – perhaps I didn't understand – if so, couldn't someone, anyone, talk to me and help me understand?. I also kept remembering Norman's request to be treated as one of my horses. Well, for sure, my horses had always received better medical and nursing care than Norman had and I would never have left my horses the way he had been left by the medical staff. I could not help but recognise how unfair, wrong and totally unacceptable it was but, of course, the big difference is veterinary services are privately paid for.

I did not receive a reply to my email to the Medical Director for several days which understandably annoyed me, but then he was a busy man and Norman only one patient in a large hospital. The trouble for me was that that one patient was my brother.

During my visit to Norman the next day he was still very down. The hospital staff were much more amenable and I tried to explain what had gone on since Norman had been admitted. Now, Norman was easily tearful and this was the first time he said he was so scared, which remained with him throughout the rest of his illness. I can only imagine being trapped in your own body as he was and, during the middle of the night, people coming to your bed and starting to push you through the corridors. It is the middle of the night and you have no idea where they are taking you, or even if your sister will find you. The majority of people as ill as Norman, with difficulty talking and communicating, would feel unnerved and afraid. The worst of all is that you are defenceless and can do nothing about it. You realise that the people who are pushing you can do anything they want to and you cannot fight back. You are at their mercy. How scary is that? The experience most certainly left its mark on Norman which remained with him.

A week later, I received an apologetic email from the Medical Director of the hospital stating that he was not at all happy with what had been said to me by the nursing staff.

He also tried to reassure me that it was not true and Norman would be looked after to the best of their ability. Incredulously, despite this diabolical start to Norman's stay in the Burns Ward, they looked after him during his stay better than any other ward, possibly due to their knowledge and understanding of moving people with extremely painful skin due to extensive burns; but – the damage was done – from now on Norman was permanently "scared" and frequently tearful. Throughout our journey, it has struck me many times how fragile our "mind" is. What seems to be a very innocent and insignificant remark results in a devastating and long-lasting condition.

I continued to visit Norman every day as before and kept well away from discussing anything to do with the Bomber Group, and I most certainly did not tell him that our uncle had passed away. I continued to push to get Norman transferred to somewhere more suitable as I genuinely thought that if he stayed in the hospital much longer he would soon become a hospital statistic. Eventually, I received a telephone call out of the blue from Admissions at a NHS Neurological Nursing Home. The manager was visiting the hospital and would like to assess Norman for a transfer to their nursing home. She was assessing four patients but only had two beds available. The manager asked what day/times I could make and I said just tell be a date and time and I will be there. After several attempts at trying to contact the nursing home (they appeared to be very busy), eventually we agreed a date and time. I asked a few questions, especially what is the carer-to-patient ratio, and she assured me that they had many more people to care for Norman than the hospital. They visited and assessed Norman and agreed to take him. I felt relieved, as he was going to be transferred to a nursing home with more staff, and better facilities. Norman would be able to have his own room with belongings, television, radio, wheelchair and, most importantly, they promised he would have physio. Norman, however, was very cynical and depressed – close to tears most of the time. He did not want to be transferred to a nursing home (which

I could understand). I told him how positive I felt about the move and he said, sarcastically, "Glad you are!". The thought crossed my mind that he may be thinking that, because the nursing home is an hour's drive away, I would not visit him so often and I reassured him that although I would not be able to visit every day I would visit him five days a week but this promise failed to reassure him. I could not help but feel pleased though, as I believed this was a step towards him recovering. We just now had to wait. Finally, the day and time we had been given came and we waited and waited and waited. Norman was beginning to get more and more agitated. A nurse eventually came into the room and said that they did not have transport and therefore the transfer has been postponed to another day (I think Norman was relieved). The next transfer date and time came and the transport arrived. Norman did not seem himself at all and I called the nurse. The nurse called a doctor who diagnosed that he had yet another urine infection and postponed the transfer. A few days later I received a telephone call to say that Norman was on his way to the nursing home. I asked if I had time to get to the hospital before they left and they said if you hurry. I did not want Norman leaving the hospital without knowing that we would be there with him. I rushed to the hospital and made it just in time to tell Norman, in person, that I would meet him at the nursing home.

Chapter 3
Nursing Home

Norman arrived at the nursing home and was transferred to a room which he shared with another patient. Sadly, Norman's roommate could hardly speak and was therefore no comfort or company to Norman. We arranged a television for him and a few bits and pieces and although Norman had never been a great one for television, after six months of no television and little radio, it was at least company for him. His roommate also had a television and it proved a challenge to only change the station on the television you wanted to and not both. Initially, when we frequently changed both televisions Norman's roommate uttered very loud noises of annoyance but no speech. We learnt to cope within a day or so, as the last thing we wanted to do was interfere with Norman's roommate who appeared to be very young but when I spoke to his family he was actually older than he looked and his adult daughter also visited him. His story was as sad as everybody's in the nursing home. He had been abroad travelling on his motorbike and had crashed sustaining brain damage. Coincidentally, an ambulance had been travelling behind him and so was immediately on the scene of the crash.

Very quickly, I learnt that everyone you spoke to in the nursing home had a very sad story to tell regarding their resident family member or friend. It was a world I had never imagined; my head had been firmly in the sand; but now I had no choice but to adapt and learn to cope.

Norman stayed in bed for a couple of days to settle in, whilst the home sorted out a wheelchair for him. I visited the next day during meal time and found one of the carers feeding him. Remembering my "telling off" in the hospital, I asked enquiringly why he wasn't feeding himself and she looked at me quizzically and said "He can't," to which, I replied, "Yes he can, but you do have to put everything in place for him and help." She said, disbelievingly, "Show me". I sat Norman up into position, set his plate in front of him, cut the food into mouth-sized pieces and handed Norman a fork with a large handle which made it easier for him to hold. He started to put the food on his fork and place the food into his mouth. The carer was clearly shocked but I have to say the message went round the nursing home like lightning and after that day Norman was positioned so that he could place a loaded fork/spoon into his mouth himself. He still could not use his left hand, only his right, and because his swallowing had been damaged by his stroke he tended to put too much food into his mouth at any one time without swallowing and so he needed to be supervised to ensure he did not choke, and to ensure he was able to scoop up the food with only one hand, but at least it was a little bit of independence.

Every time I visited, I was asked for something else, more clothing, toothpaste, shaving cream, shaver, shower gel, talc, etc. In its own way this was comforting because at least I felt that Norman was now being cared for. In the end, I learnt to "stock up" for a couple of months with everything Norman needed as their demands proved to be quite time consuming when I tried to fit it in with working full time, visiting Norman, and my own life. Very early on I was invited to "meet the team". It was an introductory meeting with Norman, myself, Kevin, the doctor, nursing staff, physio, etc. They said that it was a fact finding meeting for Norman's benefit. The truth was, it was a fact finding exercise for the staff to learn about Norman's visitors and family members so that they could assess who they would be dealing with in addition to Norman. No further meetings were held, no specific changes to Norman's benefit were made and I began to realise that Norman had been right. His tears when told he was to be transferred to a nursing home were justified!

Friends of Norman had commented to me that it was very likely that he would become "institutionalised". The nursing home was an institution but it was not Norman or I that became "institutionalised" – it was everybody that worked there, and in order to "fit in" and cope, we had no option but to adjust!

For all of us, the first week was very difficult trying to make the adjustments needed. Travelling alone was now 2 to 2½ hours a day for me after a day's work, and the demands the nursing home put onto its patient's relations were also greater. Washing of clothes was a big issue with staff pushing families to take the washing home but the facility was there for patients' clothing to be washed which I chose. The challenge here was that all clothing had to be named and, even when named, frequently went missing so constant demands were made for new clothing (often the clothing was sitting in the laundry room unsorted). Clothing was difficult for Norman due to his height. Carers wanted "easy" clothing such as jogging bottoms – the problem was I couldn't find extra-long jogging bottoms so Norman's trousers often came to just past his knee – especially after a few washes at high temperature causing them to shrink. He was never one to be over particular about his appearance but, understandably, he was not too amused at his hairy legs from the knees down being on display!

However, within a couple of days Norman was allocated a wheelchair and he was no longer bed-ridden. His daily routine now was to have breakfast, be washed and dressed, and be placed into his wheelchair. Norman had been transferred to the nursing home in early June and we were blessed with a very good summer. We arrived within a couple of days and found him sitting in his wheelchair; it was so good to see him sitting up. His room was on the first floor and the residents were all pushed out to a hallway and lined up in front of a large television. This upset Norman big-time. He was the only one who could talk slightly at that time and he felt surrounded by "abnormal" and "scary" people. It distressed him deeply to be "one of them" and it distressed me to arrive and see Norman lined up in a corridor so upset. His face would light up when he saw me and he was very anxious for me to take him away from this environment if only for an hour or two.

A huge benefit though was that we were able to push Norman outside into fresh air and find our way round the grounds. In order to get out one had to negotiate the numeric locks and lift which certainly cured me of my silly fear of lifts! My ability to manoeuvre a heavy wheelchair had to improve. Now on the ground floor, we asked reception where we could go and they directed us to the "chickens". This was a very small area of grass where the staff kept three chickens and as I started to push Norman, out of the blue he said "I'm having a wee", to which I replied, "Too much information", but smiled inwardly whilst thinking how strange it must be for him and I guess part of him coming to terms with the situation was to mention it out loud. A small shelter had been erected and some chairs lived around the grassy area. It was very pleasant, but soon became quite claustrophobic as this was the only outside area to take your relations to. Still, for our first outing with Norman in his wheelchair, it made an enormous change to the hospital ward and the weather was glorious. It was time to take Norman back and I asked where I should leave him, they directed me to a communal area where a couple of other patients were sitting asleep in front of the television. I took Norman in there and said goodbye and to this day I can still hear him – near to tears he said "Is that it – are you just going to leave me here?" Unless you experience it, I do not think anyone can understand the helplessness of leaving a person who is now completely helpless themselves and reliant upon others for everything in a nursing home. It was heart-breaking and I left choking back tears myself and this is one of the many experiences that has burnt itself into my memory for life.

It was now quite a trek to visit Norman but I had promised him that I would be there four or five days a week. Luckily, initially, I still had holiday left and so took half days only on Tuesday and Thursday. When my holiday ran out, I approached my employers and asked if I could shorten my day by two hours which meant I could leave work at 2 pm and get to the nursing home by 3.30 pm to see Norman. My employers were extremely supportive showing incredible compassion and willingly agreed. I recognise that few employers would be as good as they were and will always be grateful to them for their understanding as it was an enormous help.

I arrived one day to see Norman and he was still quite miserable. The curtain was drawn dividing his part of the room to his roommate and trying to cheer Norman up a carer put her head through the curtains and said "Boo." Norman laughed and it was good to see, but I did not realise how this small and innocent gesture to cheer him up was going to escalate.

The next routine started to establish itself, visit Norman Monday, Wednesday, Friday, Saturday and Sunday. If his meal was ready, I would help him to eat it. He hated the home and wanted to go out as much as possible so I would push his wheelchair around the grounds for an hour or more to the amusement of many of the staff and visitors as I re-entered the building dripping wet from perspiration (I think I became the in-house entertainment – but it was good for my weight!). The grounds were quite small and Norman hated being still in his wheelchair so we just went round and round the same place. To the chickens, back to outside the hospital building, up the drive, back to the Lawns building over to Jaeger building back to the chickens, into Jaeger building for a coffee and repeat. At least my fitness improved! The nursing home was near to Stansted airport and so planes flew over the grounds regularly. Norman loved planes but his passion was for World War II planes, not today's planes. Nevertheless, it still proved to be a welcome distraction and something to comment upon.

One day, bored with the regular circle, I decided to take Norman down the drive, along the roadside and back into the nursing home via their side gate. This idea appealed to Norman because he actually made it out into the real world. Whilst pushing his wheelchair along the path, suddenly it veered off the path into the kerb of the road. What a lesson this was. We had come to a dropped kerb way which had snatched the wheelchair and I simply was not strong enough to hold it from running down the slope of the footpath into the road. Luckily no vehicles were being driven down the road, otherwise we would not be here to tell the tale. I fully recognised the danger of this encounter and perhaps looking for someone else to blame other than my own stupidity I wondered why one did not have a health and safety lesson pushing a wheelchair before taking a patient out of the nursing home.

Gradually now, when I arrived to see Norman he greeted me with "Boo." Initially it was funny but it began to snowball. Eventually, I asked Norman to say "Hello" or "Hi" – not "Boo." We were thinking of taking him out to meet his friends and I was very conscious of their reaction if he greeted them with "Boo." As we approached people whilst I was pushing Norman around the grounds, he would say "Boo" but he did stop when I asked him to. Then, one Friday, to my horror and dismay as a carer came out of one of the buildings they greeted Norman with "Boo." I glared at them in disbelief of what I had just heard and moved on to another building and then – can you believe it – yet another carer came out of that building and greeted Norman with "Boo." I was shocked, angered and disgusted, that the carers should approach Norman a 64-year-old man in this way. To me, it was far from helping a severely ill person to recover. I was so angry but managed to keep my cool as I took Norman back to his room and went to find the person in charge. We had a reasonably long chat during which, although I was extremely polite, I could not disguise the tone in my voice due to both anger and distress. I found out that Norman had now been "nicknamed" Boo and everyone in the nursing home – and visitors – called him Boo. She said – "That was Norman." I made it clear that he never said "Boo" before being admitted and told her about the carer innocently putting her head round the curtains and saying "Boo." I also made it clear that it needed to change from this moment forward and to give her her due she said "What you are saying is that you want your brother spoken to with the respect of a 64-year-old man and not a child." I looked at her and said "Yes." She said that she would do her best but asked for me to correct anyone calling Norman "Boo" in my presence which naturally I agreed to. A few of the carers fought this and challenged me basically laughing saying "Oh, what is it I mustn't call him …?" but I was adamant that Norman was not going around saying "Boo" to everyone he met and it probably took four weeks or more for him to stop, but with some carers it remained a laughing matter in the background until the day he left.

Driving home that day, I thought about how fragile the mind is. I remembered the film that I watched several years earlier – *Escape from Colditz* – the escape committee had agreed an escape plan whereby one of the prisoners acted mentally ill at all times in the hope of being sent home. The planned worked well and he was sent home but, by then, he's acting had become real life and he was now mentally ill and damaged for life.

Norman had gone through so much, who could blame him for disappearing into a memory of a pretty female carer opening the curtains and saying "Boo" – it made him smile and laugh. Sadly, if he did not voice "Boo," but just thought it, no one would know and therefore not judge him, but he seemed to have lost that judgement.

By now Norman's roommate had changed and coincidentally the person who was next to him for a while in the hospital now shared Norman's room and they became great mates. His wife (who we had met in the hospital) mum, dad and brother, visited regularly and it almost became an extended family. Saturdays became a bit of a party day. Norman's roommate's wife and family, would visit and Norman and I joined them for a chat. Although Norman did not engage in a two-way conversation, he would answer questions – especially "Do you want a sandwich?" and Norman did enjoy sitting there listening to the chat. Also home-made sandwiches were handed round and this habit Norman readily accepted and thoroughly enjoyed. We agreed to take both Norman and his roommate out together when we visited which meant that they both benefited from extra visits, but the nursing home put a stop to this saying that we could only push our own relations out into the grounds – to this day, I do not understand why. I can only assume it was some health and safety rule but it was a shame because yet again the only people who suffered were Norman and his roommate as depending upon who visited, one was left behind. They both did however make me laugh when a day out was arranged and they both flatly refused to go without the other. Us relations heard a lot about this from the disgruntled staff – how dare inmates be disobedient and show some character! It was good to see them both despite their disabilities stand up for what they wanted and fight the institution they were in. I still smile at that today!

One Monday or Tuesday, as I was walking into the nursing home, I saw Norman's roommate's wife walking purposely towards me. Once in hearing distance she blurted out "Norman has been crying all weekend and is upsetting my husband." She also complained to the nursing home that her husband was distressed due to Norman crying. That day, when I parked Norman's wheelchair and was ready to leave he started to sob and all staff and visitors soon swarmed round him sympathising. Unfortunately, this was making him worse so I went to the wheelchair and started to push him away. "Come on Norman, we are going for another walk". Once settled I took him back and left him. The nursing home dealt with this event by transferring his roommate to another room which was a shame because they had become friends, and by prescribing Norman with antidepressants. When I said that Norman did not like taking pills they replied that it was a small dose. This prescription stayed with him until he died with side effects of being drowsy. Every pill seems to give a side effect. I had found out earlier that his "itchy back" was also a side effect. I thought to myself that I would be crying if left in the nursing home, so I must need antidepressants as well!

Opposite the nursing home was a pub and I heard talk about some patients being taken there from time to time. I hate pubs but both Norman and Kevin were only too keen to go. So Kevin came with me that Saturday and we gave Norman a few choices of where he could go. He answered "Pub." Now we needed to learn the best way to negotiate the road with a wheelchair. We coped easily, and it became a regular occurrence. It was so good to see Norman respond to being in not only a normal environment but one he was familiar with and comfortable in. We were so lucky with the weather as the summer continued to be back-to-back sunshine so we sat out in their gardens and I watched Norman "people watching". The wasps were challenging, especially around Norman, but no one was stung. One day it poured with rain and we tried to get Norman inside but had to give up as the pub was not wheelchair friendly with respect to width of doors and corridors.

The weeks had now found another routine. Visit Norman Monday, Wednesday, Friday, Saturday and Sunday. The first question he always asked me was "Where's my sandwich?" It was good to see him eat it. He still hated being in the nursing home with a passion, so it was my task to get him out into the grounds as quickly as possible and push him around. Saturday and Sunday, Kevin came and we took Norman over to the pub. Seeing the difference in Norman at the pub prompted me to think about how I could get him out and about a bit more. Someone mentioned to me cars which had been adapted to take wheelchairs and so I started to look into this. Norman mentioned Duxford Air Show which was coming up and I promised to get him there one way or another. I spoke to the nursing home and they said that they would do their best as "family days" were sometimes arranged, but they would not promise. However they would not entertain taking Norman's roommate and, again, I do not understand why.

Meanwhile my research into wheelchair accessible cars proved successful and I arranged for one to be driven to the nursing home from Wales for Norman's approval. Norman being a "big chap" always had big cars. This car was a Kia people carrier which had been converted to take four passengers plus a wheelchair. The wheelchair sat in between the two back seats and so the disabled person was with the passengers – not in the boot. Norman said he liked it so we bought it – just in time to take him to Duxford. However, the nursing home came up trumps and said that their driver Dan would take Norman and us to Duxford. The downside was that we had to drive past Duxford (it was half way from us to the nursing home) to get to the nursing home as they refused to meet us there. This day was so successful. We saw a totally different Norman as we pushed him around the event. Norman did not feel "dressed" unless he was carrying his camera. We had brought his camera with us and placed it on his lap and I wallowed in his smile. The camera was now far too heavy for him to hold and use but clearly he felt "whole" now that it sat on his lap. His friends were there from the Bomber Group and Sally B and they all came up to him and made a huge fuss of him – more smiles – great! Norman had been their unofficial photographer, fundraiser and committee member. One friend in particular was sitting in the front seat of his car on oxygen. Dan said quietly to us that Norman's friend at this point in time was more at risk than Norman. As we watched them together, it was very clear that they both were enjoying their time together immensely. We decided to take Norman around the site and pushed his wheelchair into a hangar which he had been into many, many times. It had a ramp up onto a mezzanine floor and back down again. It was very busy and people towered over Norman in his wheelchair. Suddenly, he started to recite "Boo Boo Boo". I was shocked, as this was a repetition of what had gone on during his early days of being transferred to the nursing home. We looked for the shortest route out from the hangar and pushed Norman out as quickly as possible. Once out into the open, away from the people, he settled and stopped saying "Boo". Another lesson for us in how fragile he was.

That day, it poured with rain but we managed to keep Norman dry. He devoured several of his favourite sandwich –

beef - and chips disappeared as did a couple of glasses of beer. I was in awe of how Dan dealt with all aspects of Norman's care that day – he was so incredibly firm, yet compassionate and respectful. It was like an apprenticeship for us, we learnt so much from Dan on how to cope with a severely disabled person. I admired Dan greatly, for his total kindness, patience, empathy, and understanding, of disabled people. He liked Norman and Norman liked him and it showed. To this day, I look back on Duxford as one of the most special days – not only for Norman but for us as we learnt so much and were given the confidence to take Norman out on our own. The difference in the way Dan communicated with the disabled was so obvious compared to other carers. He treated them as normal human beings suffering from an illness, not as "idiots" which other carers seemed to do, but at the same time he was firm when needed and would not allow Norman to put too much food into his mouth without swallowing first – another invaluable lesson for us for the future. Dan actually said one day to a young carer "Norman has achieved more in his lifetime than you will ever do." Dan is the person I remember throughout this journey with the most admiration and respect.

It was now September and the nights were drawing in and the days not so hot. We could no longer use the pub across the road as it was too cold to sit outside. We had purchased the wheelchair accessible car which allowed us the flexibility to take Norman out and about ourselves. We started to take Norman to different pubs to see which was the most suitable. Eventually, we tried a pub by the railway station. The owner and barmaid could not have been more accommodating or nicer to Norman. They spoilt him rotten. The routine was to take Norman there Tuesday, Thursday and sometimes at weekends, although we tended to only go on the days that they were not watching football or rugby as we did not want to be in their way. Before long, the other regulars in the pub recognised us and started to chat. Nobody ignored Norman because he was in a wheelchair and they all spoke to him like a normal human being and not an idiot which was so important. We mentioned Norman's passion for photographing WWII aeroplanes and they encouraged us to take some of his photos in which we were more than happy to do. Three chaps came over and started to look at the photos and chat to Norman. The barmaid brought Norman cheese and biscuits every time and he started to look for them. Norman could still use his right hand slightly to eat but not his left and the barmaid insisted he used his left. She would tap his right hand and say "No, use your left"; he would laugh and attempt to use his left. She proved to be a good physio as Norman took notice of her but not us. If he spilt his drink or dropped the cheese and biscuits, the barmaid smiled and cleared it up. It was no problem.

Witnessing the difference of seeing Norman in the nursing home compared to out of the nursing home made me start to think more and more of how I could discharge him. He had been fortunate enough to make sufficient money from his own business so, at least, money should not be an issue. He continued to be extremely unhappy and desperate to get out of the nursing home and live with us. His two-bedroom bungalow was far too small and our own house was also too small. I discussed with Norman the possibility of selling both properties and buying a larger house to accommodate him, a carer, Kevin and I. Norman was very positive about it and even told Terence and Connor, his ex-business partner and colleague. I was surprised to hear that Norman had blurted this out to Terence and Connor the next time they visited because their visit was a while after we had discussed it. I spoke to the nursing home and they could see no reason why he should not be discharged. He would need a lot of equipment and support, but it could be done.

One day, whilst searching on my mobile phone, I came across a four-bedroom house just a mile down the road from where we lived. Kevin and I arranged a viewing. The house seemed perfect for Norman. Just inside the front door was the dining room which was large enough to convert into a hospital bedroom and wet room. The remainder of the downstairs consisted of a large wide hallway leading into a spacious kitchen which led into a generous living room and conservatory. Apart from the bedroom adaptations and widening one doorway the living area downstairs was ideal for manoeuvring a large, heavy, wheelchair. Entry proved a little more difficult as the front door led straight into a porch and a second front door. The back entrance was along the garden leading to two large steps to the back door. The back door led into a narrow utility area not suitable for a wheelchair. Ideally though, the conservatory had French doors leading onto the garden. The drop from the French doors was at least two feet BUT the plan was to lay a patio at the height of the conservatory with wheelchair access from the front of the house along the side of the conservatory on to the patio and into the house via the French doors – perfect!

The front of the house was laid to concrete with a shared concrete drive leading to the back of the house with more concrete which led to the back garden. The whole outside of the house was extremely wheelchair friendly. The location was just one mile from Norman's bungalow so we were in the same area for the local pub and friends. We asked the sellers if we could bring Norman and naturally they agreed. I couldn't wait to tell Norman on my next visit. We piled him into the car and drove him from the nursing home to the house. Sadly we were unable to get him into the house but he was able to see the outside and we described the inside and our plans. I told him that it would cost slightly more than what we would sell both our existing properties for. He accepted this willingly as, at last, there was a plan for him to escape from *Colditz* – whoops – sorry – the nursing home.

I had met Norman's financial advisor a week or two earlier and arranged a meeting with him, Norman, myself and Kevin. We met him outside the nursing home and agreed to take Norman to our favourite pub by the railway. We loaded Norman into the newly acquired access vehicle and off we went. The meeting went well and it was agreed to make an offer on the house.

Within a couple of days I spoke to the manager at the nursing home and explained what we intended to do. She felt that there was no reason for Norman not to be discharged providing all the necessary facilities were put in place. It was felt prudent to arrange for their Occupational Therapist to visit the house to assess what adaptations needed to be made, as if they did not meet the required criteria, Norman would not be discharged. The present owners of the house were extremely helpful and agreed to let her visit to take the measurements needed in order to make the necessary plans. We all visited the house again, I was so grateful to the current owners – the Occupational Therapist loved the house and gave us her recommendations regarding adaptations. Everything seemed to be going in the right direction, so we made an offer on the house which was accepted and I told Norman who was delighted – it was now October.

Meanwhile, day-to-day living at the nursing home continued. The doctor had ordered Norman's catheter to be removed some time ago which had relieved me no end (but did confuse me a little bearing in mind that the hospital had refused to do this because they had diagnosed stones in his bladder which needed to be removed by an operation). Urine infections did not seem to happen so often and Norman's health appeared to improve slightly. However, despite knowing that we were arranging to discharge him, mentally he was declining and, to some degree, I could understand this. One day, on arrival at the nursing home, Norman was not sitting in the corridor and so I asked where he was. When I found him, he was sitting next to a carer who was encouraging him to colour an elephant – pink! Another time I arrived he was being asked to make flowers out of paper. Although, I understood the reasons behind these activities, for Norman who was a very intelligent and studious person it was degrading and not "him" one little bit. Remembering the time when I arrived and I was told that Norman was attending the multiple-choice quiz is much more pleasurable and rewarding. I walked into the room and he looked up to acknowledge me and I asked him if he wished to go outside (in the past he couldn't wait), this day he asked to go out after the quiz had finished. His general knowledge was still extremely good and he surprised everyone present. Naturally, he answered more questions than anyone else in the room – that was the Norman I knew!

Having the mobility car allowed us much more freedom. It was now October/November and the weather wasn't too good, so we decided to take Norman out for lunch on Sunday to the local pub to his bungalow. It was an hour's drive from the nursing home to the pub, lunch, and an hour's drive back. As we pushed Norman into the pub, we were welcomed by a few old friends of his who came up to him and made a big fuss of him. Shook his hand, bought him half a pint of shandy, and made even more fuss of him. It was great to see him laugh and smile – such a different Norman to the one the nursing home saw.

Meanwhile back at the neurological nursing home, they were being very difficult and obstructive regarding Norman's discharge and the purchase of the house and so a General Power of Attorney was raised and given to them so that I could continue. Norman was being subjected to mental capacity test after mental capacity test and Kevin and I were summoned to attend a meeting to discuss his discharge. There were probably ten people from the nursing home there. Not long into the meeting, I felt interrogated – one question I will never forget "So you are expecting a better standard of living for yourselves are you?" I remained calm and said it was my intention for all members of the new household, Norman, Norman's live-in carer, Kevin and myself and even the dog, to enjoy the best life possible when taking into consideration the difficulties we were all going to face coping with Norman's serious and extensive care needs. The meeting ended with my shackles well and truly up – not for the first time and, sadly, not for the last time either.

The nursing home continued to constantly subject Norman to mental capacity tests. When I arrived at the nursing home, Norman would greet me, immediately, with "I'm an idiot." I replied "You are not", but he insisted he was an idiot. I asked why and he could not tell me. He also kept saying "I'm scared" which related back to the episode in the Burns Ward at the hospital. I told him he was not and he asked "Why not?" I replied "You are my big brother, seriously ill, but whilst you remain my big brother, you will never be an idiot because I won't allow it". Although trying to reassure him, I was bemused and then, finally, I realised he was being given mental capacity test after mental capacity test and being told that he had failed. No matter how many tests the nursing home subjected him to and despite his serious disabilities in recalling words and pronouncing them – he never faltered – he wanted to come home and live with us.

Early one Thursday evening, I received a telephone call from the nursing home and naturally was initially worried why they were calling. Thankfully, Norman was absolutely fine but they were calling because he had failed one of their mental capacity tests and a "Best Interests" meeting was being called to which I needed to attend. To me, this was yet another obstruction to his discharge. I asked what the questions were he had failed on and I was told that he had been asked by the Occupational Therapist who had visited the new house its price and had given an amount which was obviously far too low. The second question was: "What is the address of the new house?" and he could only give the name of the village - not the full address. A day and time for the meeting was arranged and the telephone conversation ended. As soon as I put the receiver down, I was livid. I had only told Norman the difference from selling his bungalow and our house and buying the new house which was exactly the sum Norman had told the Occupational Therapist. In addition, because the new house was only a mile down the road from his current bungalow and did not have a number only a house name, I had not told Norman the full address – just the village name which again was the answer he had given. Both questions he had answered correctly and yet told that he had failed. To me this fell little short of mental cruelty. The person asking the questions did not only NOT know the answers but, in my opinion, they were overstepping the mark with a view to privileged information. The meeting date came and immediately the meeting convened I made it very clear how disgusted I was that they should fail Norman on giving correct answers to questions asked that they themselves did not know the answers to and, in addition, the said questions were way out of line being an invasion of privacy especially as I had given them a copy of the General Power of Attorney. The General Power of Attorney had been raised in October 2013 specifically to enable me to act on Norman's behalf to purchase the house. It would be superseded once the Lasting Power of Attorney for Property & Financial affairs had been registered which would be January 2014 (after completion of purchase). The neurological nursing home was not familiar with a General Power of Attorney and continued to subject Norman to mental capacity tests. Yet again, the damage was done. Norman felt he was an idiot and scared. Understandably, I felt particularly stressed being continually subjected to obstacles being put in my way regarding his discharge and I decided to ring a solicitor and discuss this with him. He told me that the nursing home had no authority to refuse discharge. The matter could be referred to the courts to decide but the court's decision would likely be that it is in Norman's best interests to be cared for at home. The battle continued!

During December, whilst visiting Norman, the Manager of the nursing home came up to me and said that when Norman arrived he had been put in a room share and she had promised that he would be transferred to his own room as soon as one came free. I was a little surprised at this as we were three months into his discharge. Norman wasn't keen on moving but I said "Well let's go and look at it". The room was in another building to where Norman was currently. So for him it was quite a big thing as it was a complete change of people and surroundings he had come to know and looking back I think I gave insufficient consideration to these two factors, forgetting how fragile Norman was mentally. I pushed him across to the other building and to his proposed room. It was quite a large room, obviously with its own ensuite, large window with not a fantastic view for him simply because we were on the first floor. We agreed to Norman being moved within a couple of days and I was surprised to learn how different the running of each building was when it was managed by the same people. For instance, the first building tended to use pads to manage incontinence, whilst the second building used convenes. Norman was suffering from sore private parts and the first building dealt with this by ordering a special cushion for his wheelchair whilst the second building coped with it by keeping him in bed for 22 hours per day which I am convinced compromised his rheumatoid arthritis and general neuropathy.

Within a few visits, I was with Norman in his room when two carers arrived to carry out personal care. Immediately, Norman screamed at full lung capacity. I was thoroughly bemused as this was all new behaviour to me. I asked him why he was screaming and to stop. He did. The carers made a move towards him and he screamed again. This carried on until I was told to leave and escorted outside the room.

Outside I could hear Norman screaming at full lung capacity like a wild animal being tortured and remembered back to the hospital when he was intolerant of the patient screaming in the side ward next to him. This behaviour simply was not Norman and, naturally, upset me a great deal and I could not understand the nursing home's reaction. Seeing I was upset, a carer came to talk to me and said that he struggled to cope with Norman now as he screamed so loudly in his ear. I went to the office and spoke to the nurse on duty. Basically, they just accepted it, and I was shown to the waiting room. I was shocked, bemused, traumatised, coupled to every other emotion you could imagine. Dan saw me and recognised how distressed I was and came to sit with me. He was the driver for the nursing home's minibus and had accompanied us on the family day when we took Norman to Duxford air show. I had so much respect for Dan as his empathy and caring for people so stricken with such a disgusting illness was faultless. He had been such a strength to us teaching us how to cope with Norman's disabilities. Clearly, he felt for both Norman and I now and gave me his home and mobile telephone numbers saying do not hesitate to contact him at any time should we need his help or guidance after discharging Norman. He is the one person from the nursing home I shall always remember with fondness.

Norman continued to scream at full lung capacity for 25 minutes until personal care was completed. It echoed throughout the whole of the first floor of the care home. For me, it was completely inhuman. I understood that his convene/pads needed to be changed – but could they not hear how upset Norman was. Why did they inflict their will upon him in such an inhumane way?

Again, I went to the office and spoke to those on duty. They told me that Norman had started to scream at the other building just before he was transferred to this building and they considered it to be "learnt behaviour". *Really*!? They said in case it was pain they had prescribed paracetamol and anti-depressants. This still upsets me today. Something happened. This behaviour was so out of character for Norman. Throughout his life he had been non-confrontational, **never** making a fuss or nuisance of himself. There was a reason for Norman to scream like this. It coincided with the nursing home keeping him in bed for 22 hours. He suffered from rheumatoid arthritis coupled to general neuropathy. Did they not realise how stiff and frozen his joints would be? Did they not realise how painful neuropathy is? Did they not know that paracetamol is completely ineffective against rheumatoid arthritis pain? The nursing home certainly showed no empathy for Norman being "scared" and feeling "an idiot". To this day, I think it is horrendous to inflict your will on someone in such a way – just imagine you have been lying in bed for 22 hours – you are stiff and sore:-

The doors open. There is nothing you can do. You can not move. You can not run. You cannot escape. You cannot shake your arm or lift a leg. You cannot resist. You cannot fight. You are 100% defenceless. You can scream. Nobody listens. Two people impose their wish upon you. They lay you flat. They turn you. You try to say that you cannot tolerate the pain being turned on your side. You cannot pronounce the words. You can pronounce "F… Off". You try that. They don't listen. You try to say "My knee, my knee." They don't care. You are turned one way, then the other. You try to say "My joints, my muscles." They don't care. They don't listen. You try to say, "I'm going to fall I'm too close to the edge." They don't care. They don't listen. Finally, the torturous ordeal is over. You are exhausted from screaming. You are exhausted by the fear, pain and fatigue, you suffer. But they have gone . . . until the next time!

For me, the nearest descriptive word is "rape". Two people enforcing their will upon you in a personal manner. I never condoned anybody ignoring Norman's screaming. I took it very seriously indeed and I do not believe that reassuring Norman helped at all. Screaming remained an issue in the discharge process and continued to be recorded and reported upon but nobody did anything – it was just accepted – it was Norman. My point of view – no it wasn't! How could it be Norman when he had not started to scream until enduring five months in hospital and six months in a nursing home – twelve months after collapsing – something had changed.

Whilst Norman was at home, we did manage to control his screaming but we never cured it completely and never understood it completely. It became clear that Norman was unable to tell us what the problem was and it was left to observation and educated guesswork. A couple of years after his death I was talking to someone who had neuropathy in the lower part of their leg and she said "Nobody has any understanding how painful this is," and I asked "Surely your doctor does and/or the specialist?" and she replied "They do not have a clue of the extent of the pain," and my mind went straight back to Norman. He had general neuropathy coupled to rheumatoid arthritis coupled to speech difficulties caused by a stroke caused by the hospital leaving a catheter in from January to April, causing sepsis, coupled to cognitive impairment caused by his brain disease and stroke resulting in him not being able to recall words easily and pronounce them – no wonder he screamed – no wonder he was scared – surely we could have done more! I believe the knowledge is out there somewhere, it is just so difficult to tap into. In my opinion, the medical and care professionals should be ashamed of themselves.

Sometime during Norman's illness he had said that he wanted a "big black dog" and I decided to buy a black Labrador as I thought it would give Norman something to focus on and hopefully help him to recover. I did not want a puppy as I wanted a dog Norman could pat, and I found Jet a "small" black Labrador. Even his name made us smile as it was quite apt for Norman with his love of planes. Jet was the pick of the litter and still with the owner of his dad. We went to visit Jet and fell for him immediately such a soft and amenable little chap. He was still kept in a kennel and although handled had not been house-trained. We arranged to bring Jet home and I couldn't wait to show Norman.

During our next visit Jet came with us. Kevin stayed in the car with Jet and I rushed up stairs to tell Norman. I started to push Norman to the car whilst saying to him that I had a surprise for him. We got to the car and he saw Jet and a big smile spread across his face – such a rare occasion now. Jet was still tiny and sat on Norman's lap. It wasn't long before the news of Jet spread around the nursing home and carers asked to see Jet. I said "But what happens if he does a wee?" – the reply was "We will clear it up." "Fab. Ok I'll go and get him." This day, Norman was already in bed and the carers encouraged me to put Jet on his bed. Jet is such a gorgeous dog he went to sleep with Norman's hand resting on him. This is one of the days I remember with such affection and can't help but smile. Jet has proved himself to be an adorable dog, the carers were fantastic and Norman had something to love.

A couple of weeks later Norman asked if I was going to sell Jet and he seemed upset. I replied "No, why?" and he said that one of the carers had told him that he wouldn't have Jet much longer. I never got to the bottom of this but it left me wondering what someone had said to Norman – were they joking or being cruel? Whichever it was, it was another example of how fragile Norman was.

Come December 2013, the new house was bought and we moved into it with Jet. The first task was to start the process of discussing the adaptations with the named builders for this type of work on the local Council's list as all work had to be approved. Meanwhile, my next challenge was how do we get Norman into the house? I started to research ramps and, yet again, this was new territory for me but proved to be a fairly easy challenge thanks to the internet. Ramps bought; we collected Norman from the nursing home and brought him back to the new house for the first of many Sunday lunches. "Elbows in" was the phrase for the day. Up the ramps, through the first front door, across the porch which was now covered with plywood to make it the same level, and through the second front door, down the hall which was sufficiently wide enough, into the kitchen, sharp left into the conservatory and straight into the lounge. Park the wheelchair next to our chairs in front of the television and introduce Norman to Jet. Job well done! Norman was visiting his new home. We gave Norman one of Jet's toys and encouraged him to throw it. The toy travelled a few inches and we all laughed at his pathetic throw. Still, most importantly, Norman's first visit to his new home was a great success, especially as we gave him lunch as well. We brought him home for that Christmas and every Sunday from that day until the day we finally managed to discharge him at the end of March.

On arrival during one of my visits to the nursing home, I found that Norman's wheelchair had been changed. I knew this because the footplates did not work – you could not fix them up. It made it very difficult and dangerous to load him into the car because the only way to do this was to lean the wheelchair dangerously far back in order to get his feet high enough to clear the ramp. The pressure on my back and arms to do this was enormous and took all of my strength to hold the wheelchair with him in it. I asked at the office to whom I should talk to about this and was pointed to the person responsible for the wheelchairs. She listened to me but, alas, nothing was done despite the health and safety issues endangering both Norman and myself. She did however comment that Norman would have a different wheelchair on discharge. We continued to struggle with the wheelchair but luckily no harm was done.

It was now early January 2014 and time to start the adaptations to the new house. The builder visited and measured the dining room which was to become Norman's hospital bedroom. Part of the room needed to be partitioned off for a wet room. The Occupational Therapist (OT) from the nursing home had visited earlier in the process and had said everything was OK but now I was being told that if the wet room did not meet specification, Norman would not be discharged. I decided the way forward was to arrange an on-site meeting between the builder, nursing home's OT and myself with the intention of obtaining the agreement of all involved on the day to ensure there would be no problems in discharging. The meeting day came and the builder's OT also came meaning the meeting now consists of the builder, nursing home's OT, builder's OT and me.

All hell was let loose! The builder's OT started to rant and rave that the room was nowhere near big enough. The two OTs got together and said that although Norman did not use a toilet at the nursing home, one should be included in his wet room. I could see their point and so agreed which meant the builder had to re-measure and re-do his plans. By now, the nursing home's OT (being easily led) was also ranting and raving as well saying it would not work – to which I replied "But you said it was OK". I was now feeling more than a little disconcerted and worried – had I bought a house to which Norman would not be discharged to? I approached the builder (who had escaped to another room) and said "Your OT is ranting and raving saying that the room is not large enough and cannot be converted". He rolled his eyes, sighed and mumbled "OTs" as he turned to go and talk to her. I'm left thinking – what have I done?! Recovering, I went back to the room and announced to everyone "Norman is coming home and all of you are going to make this work!" I then started to remove the few things that were on the floor and told those present that we are going to put templates on the floor so that we have a visual guide to how the room was going to be converted. The OT from the nursing home was immediately on my side and that is exactly what we did. Everything fitted in well. Still determined to make her mark, the builder's OT came in and said "It will not work because there is no room for wardrobes – where are you going to put his clothes?" Body language – I moved closer to her, looked her straight in the eyes, and said "Trivia," she repeated "It won't work you have no wardrobe" – my reply "Trivia," she stated the same again and I replied again "Trivia." She gave up and the meeting came to a close leaving me feeling more than a little drained and frazzled.

Four to six weeks later, the conversions were nearly completed and I was informed that the local social services OT now needed to visit and OK the wet room (yep – the third OT) before Norman could be discharged. You can imagine how nervous I was of his visit. The day of his visit came. He was a young chap, quiet and professional. To my delight and surprise, he complimented me on the room saying that he had rarely seen such a well-planned, good example, of a wet room (which now also housed drawers and one wardrobe for Norman's clothing). What planet was the builder's OT on?

During one of my visits to Norman about this time I was informed that, as part of the discharge process, he had to be taken out into the community to see how he coped. This was beyond my comprehension as he was never going to have to cope on his own in the community as between one and two carers had to accompany him. He needed to be pushed everywhere as he could not manoeuvre the wheelchair himself. He needed to be transported anywhere by the converted mobility vehicle, but I had learnt not to argue so I said, "OK where are you taking him?" They replied "Shopping" to which I inwardly laughed thinking that they did not know Norman very well. I could not help myself and replied "Well you won't achieve anything there, he hated shopping when he was well, let alone now. If I were you I would take him to the local pub, half a pint of shandy and something light and easy for him to eat." For the only time in the whole process they listened to me and took him to the local pub where he could "people watch" and listen to conversations – record-breaking news – he passed!

I was disappointed that the builders could not complete earlier than the end of February, but also fully aware of my struggle to get Norman discharged before then anyway. I was now told that Norman needed to be assessed for "NHS Continuing Healthcare Funding". I asked why as he was fully funded now in the nursing home but the reply was "He needs to be assessed before he can be discharged." As I have said earlier, I had learnt that it is a waste of breath to argue and so accepted it but also reminded them that, no matter what, he was coming home as soon as the adaptations were completed. I was also told around this time by the nursing home that Norman would not be eligible for NHS Continuing Healthcare because he would not score a "priority" or two "severe". My focus was firmly on getting Norman home which is what he wanted and he had never faltered, despite being continuously asked by the nursing home, so I started to make enquiries regarding carers – another blank page for me to fill. Despite asking several people at the nursing home, and the social care worker involved, I was left to carry out my own research on the internet. I found what appeared to be a suitable Care Company. I duly rang to speak to a member of their staff and they informed me that they needed to visit Norman at the nursing home to assess his care needs. I understood this and so arranged a meeting date and time with them.

The meeting time was 3 p.m. and the day came. I had arranged to take time of work and made my way to the nursing home. On arrival, I asked if the representative from the Care Company had arrived and she had not, which was OK as I was a little early. I made my way to Norman's room as the meeting was to be held in front of him. Four o'clock came and went, 5 o'clock and no representative. Naturally, I'm ringing to see if she is still coming and I am told she is. Finally, she arrives and we start the meeting to discuss Norman's care needs with Norman present and representatives from the nursing home. It was a lengthy and tedious meeting with plenty of paperwork to be completed. I could see Norman fatiguing and, as always, felt concerned. Eventually the meeting was completed and the Care Company's representative made her way home to start the process of appointing a live-in carer and I too made my way home which enabled Norman to get the rest he now desperately needed. I had become immune to being left waiting and waiting throughout this process. At least this journey has improved my patience and tolerance levels (or perhaps not!). I told myself (yep! I'm now talking to myself) I must be positive – hopefully this was a huge step forward. Shortly, Norman would have his own carer appointed and be discharged home.

Meantime, the nursing home informed me of the date and time for the local social worker to visit both Norman and myself on separate occasions. He wanted to see Norman in the nursing home and visit the home to where he was going to be discharged to. They also informed me of the date for the NHS Continuing Healthcare meeting.

For a couple of weeks, the old routine was re-established, visiting Norman during the week and bringing him home for lunch on Sundays. Sundays were proving to be extremely time-consuming due to the travelling but it was all worthwhile for Norman to have dinner in his new home and to see Jet. It worried me a little, as at times he seemed very unsettled and seemed to want to get back to the nursing home. I asked him several times if he was going to be happy living here and he never hesitated to reply with a definite "Yes." Although unable to express it, I think he was aware of my length of day.

By now, Norman had been allocated a new wheelchair which was too wide for him and he constantly slipped as there were no supports to stop him and he was unable to hold his own sitting balance. The handles were set very wide apart which made it extremely awkward to push, as you lost strength due to your arms being held so widely apart reducing the power of your shoulders. This particular day, Norman had slipped left and was literally hanging out of the wheelchair. He was at home with us at this time and although the relevant doors had been widened for a wheelchair, this particular one was much wider than his last. Kevin and I were struggling to straighten Norman as, at this stage, we did not have a hoist or any other equipment so, unfortunately, it was a case of man-handling him until we had him straight enough in the wheelchair to enable us to manoeuvre him out of the house and into the mobility car. I cannot tell you how nerve-wracking this was. Anyway we managed and drove Norman safely back to the nursing homing.

The new wheelchair was especially difficult to manoeuvre due to its extra width in the mobility car and one Sunday on arrival back to the nursing home, I started to unload Norman but the straps holding the wheelchair in place did not release properly and as I withdrew the wheelchair out of the car they snatched and pulled at it. The wheelchair is now positioned with one of its wheels off the ramp of the mobility car to the right. The straps are fully extended and cannot be released. Norman is screaming. It is 4-ish in the afternoon, dark, wet and nobody to be seen in the nursing home's car park. Norman continues to scream and scream and I add to the chaos by swearing – a lot! My swearing finally registers with Norman (as generally, I don't swear) and he stops screaming to say "Stop swearing." I replied "You stop screaming and I'll stop swearing." Peace was resumed. I managed to release the wheelchair and unload Norman safe and sound. The ramp on the mobility car took the most punishment and was now bent. It is another ordeal that I will never forget but I remember it with fondness and light-heartedness of Norman telling me off and to stop swearing (reminding me of my big brov before he fell ill) but cold shivers also run down my spine when I remember this ordeal as to what could have happened and how alone you can be in a busy car park.

Once again I spoke to the people in charge of the wheelchairs regarding Norman's new chair. I explained the problems we had with him not being supported and slipping to either side and down the wheelchair. I also explained the difficulties in getting him into the mobility vehicle as it was too wide and that it was also too wide and cumbersome to manoeuvre around the new house despite our having already widened the relevant door. Yet again, it all fell on deaf ears, the only advice I received was "Change the mobility car" – "Pardon, are you serious?" Yes they were!

Eventually someone told me about Mark, the chap that came in once or twice a week to look at the wheelchairs. Whilst walking outside one day, he was pointed out to me by someone who had a little bit of sympathy regarding our problem with the wheelchair. He was a very personable person, very understanding and showed great empathy for my predicament. It transpired that his wife was one of the nursing home's assessors for wheelchairs and had, in fact, assessed Norman and put forward her recommendation for the one he should be allocated. However, her recommendation had been overridden and he had been allocated the chair in question due to cost – it was a much cheaper option. Mark and his wife agreed that the wheelchair he was now using was not suitable, mainly because it offered no support and allowed him to slip to the side and down. They suggested coming out to the house in order to assess the need for the wheelchair to be manoeuvred around the house and naturally I welcomed their help and advice. Both came out quite quickly and totally understood my problems regarding the wheelchair and said they would do as much as they could.

The best they could achieve would be to persuade the nursing home to put Norman's new wheelchair into storage and go back to using his previous one. I asked about what wheelchair he would be discharged with and they said he could borrow one of theirs but I would have to take home the one allocated to him as well – so we would have two. This was no problem and he was put back into his previous wheelchair – the one with broken footplates but Mark did his best to repair it for us.

The days had passed and it was time for the NHS Continuing Healthcare Assessment to take place as well as an assessment from the local social worker. The social worker contacted me and arranged to visit the house during February. Unfortunately, the day he came he found me somewhat hostile as I had just been informed that Norman's NHS Continuing Healthcare Assessment had been cancelled for the second time and would be scheduled to a later date (they had no idea when). The social worker recorded in his report my frustration regarding the discharge date being delayed yet again. I had kept the nursing home informed regarding the adaptation works which were scheduled to be finished by the end of February so I had told Norman that we intended to get him home for the first week in March. I spoke to the nursing home and asked for a date as early as possible. One was made for early March but again cancelled. The only person to suffer was Norman and so often I had been subjected to phrases like "best interest", "duty of care" – but it was clearly evident to me that nobody cared about Norman's extended time in the nursing home and his loss of precious time at home. Finally, another date for late March was arranged and I was asked to attend.

Meanwhile, we decided to take some "pressies" to the barmaid of the local pub who had made us all so welcome over the past few months. So, we piled flowers and chocolates onto Norman's lap and pushed him into the pub for the last time. We explained that in a few days we would be discharging him and this was our last visit. They were thrilled for him and appreciated our token thank you – in fact, the publican was a little jealous as the "pressies" were for his barmaid and not him. A huge grin was on Norman's face as the barmaid came over, took the flowers and gave him a peck on the cheek. Days like this made the effort we put into Norman so worthwhile.

On the day of the Continuing Healthcare Assessment, Norman asked to attend. Understandably, he was keen to go home. As I entered the room, I noted several people present sitting around a large boardroom table with papers in front of them. The Chairperson introduced herself. I picked up the paperwork which was all new to me and asked what it was for as I could not see how it related to Norman. The Chairperson replied sharply "It's a template". I asked again as it did not relate to Norman. "It's a template." I looked around the table and there were insufficient copies available – people were sharing. The Chairperson opened the meeting and rushed through the paperwork. I was still struggling to understand the paperwork but by the third or fourth domain was beginning to learn. She graded the domains and very little was said by anybody else in the room – they appeared scared to speak. Clearly, the Chairperson was in a rush to get the assessment done and at one point asked me if I agreed, to which I replied "Nobody has explained the process to me and I am not familiar with it and so no, most definitely, I do not agree." The Chairperson then basically threatened me by saying "If you do not agree at this stage the process cannot continue and Norman will not be discharged." Yes – you are ahead of me – my shackles were well and truly up! I said, "I did not agree, would not agree, but Norman *will be* discharged on Monday." She then asked "Would you agree to continue if I record your disagreement on the file?" What choice did I have but to answer "Yes." I did not have the opportunity to read what she had put until several weeks later when I was sent a report – it was well watered down. The Chairperson found Norman to be not eligible for funding (despite him already being funded) and asked the meeting if they agreed. Nobody said a word. She closed the meeting saying that the social worker would take over and left the meeting in a hurry. I was furious. Why had they delayed Norman's discharge for a meeting which they knew was a waste of time as, clearly, they had already made their decision prior to the meeting? I knew Norman had funds over the threshold which wouldn't allow him to obtain social funding and could not see the point of allowing the social worker to review his finances when I knew the outcome. It seems to me, those concerned never see this process as being the invasion of privacy that it is. He had too much money in the bank to be eligible for social funding. I was then told that it was not the final decision as the file would be reviewed by another panel and Norman's discharge must wait for that decision. We were already six/seven months into the discharge process and they had already delayed it several weeks and I was determined that they were not going to delay his discharge for another six weeks awaiting the results of another hearing. I said firmly, "No. Norman is coming home in two days' time – Monday."

The Care Company I had chosen to supply a live-in carer for Norman had contacted me a few days previously to say that they had found a suitable carer. I had mentally "clocked" how excited they were at having found a suitable carer and it crossed my mind how peculiar this was as they must have plenty of carers on their books. We had already spoken and discussed Norman coming home on the Monday and had arranged to collect the carer from the railway station that Saturday.

Feeling battered and bruised from the meeting at the nursing home, I sat with Kevin discussing that this was our last night alone in the house. We had not had children and had spent all of our married life with only each other to worry about. Effective from tomorrow that was all going to change. A live-in carer, Norman, pop-in carers and, of course, Jet the Labrador. Life was about to change, but naively we thought it would not be too bad as we would no longer have to make the two-hour journey to the nursing home five days a week and Norman would be getting the one-to-one specialist care he needed and deserved.

Saturday came and I drove to the railway station to collect the carer. He was a tall chap at least 6'3" if not 6'4". Approximately, 30-ish, from abroad with a Labrador at home so he took to Jet immediately. The one thing I had not thought of is how much luggage he would need as he was staying with us four months – I should have cleared my car out (it's invariably a mess!). However, the carer managed to fold his limbs and climbed into the car and I squeezed his luggage in – it was a tight fit but it's surprising what you can achieve once you put your mind to it.

The plan was to take the carer to meet Norman on Sunday, bringing him home for his usual Sunday lunch, and then collect him Monday, which would give the carer a little time to settle in to his surroundings before coping with Norman. The nursing home had also insisted that I engage pop-in carers to assist the live-in carer during Norman's personal care and I had arranged this starting from Monday evening.

Sunday visit went well. Norman and the live-in carer Robin seemed to like each other and Norman was happy to know that this was his last night in the nursing home. My emotions were extremely mixed – very pleased at last after my tumultuous journey that we had finally reached the point of discharge for Norman. At times, when yet another obstruction had been put in my way, I had seriously doubted that this day would ever come. Robin and I left the nursing home saying "See you in the morning" to Norman, and went to collect the extra-wide wheelchair that had been allocated to Norman to store in our garage at home as Norman was coming home in a borrowed one from the nursing home which had been so kindly arranged by Mark.

The next morning Robin and I drove to the nursing home and found Norman waiting eagerly. The nursing home was not ready to discharge Norman and so we pushed him into the day room to await their OK. We were all waiting quietly when a nursing home carer entered and made his way straight to Norman. As the carer started to enter his personal space, Norman started to scream at full lung capacity – it was deafening. To our shock and amazement the carer said "Now Norman, I've told you before. When you feel like screaming, start to sing – la la la, do dar de de la la." My face must have been a picture – I know Robin's was. I could not believe my ears. Norman continues to scream and the nursing home carer continues to tell him to sing la la la. La la la. It was as if the nursing home carer was trying to "show off". He then looked up as though he was expecting to be congratulated but as he saw the look on my face and Robin's he sensibly decided to retreat and leave the room. I was stunned at the way they dealt with someone screaming – I felt like screaming back at the carer! Both Robin and I comforted Norman and reaffirmed to him that it would not be long now and he would be on his way home. Shortly afterwards, I was given the OK by the nursing home Manager and as I said thank you to her I became overwhelmed with tears and she recognised that I could hardly speak. We smiled and acknowledged each other and Robin started to push Norman down and into the mobility car. At last, we had made it, we were on our way home.

Chapter 4

Discharge Home – Live-In Carers

It was now 31st March 2014 and all of the adaptation works had been completed over a month ago. I still felt irritated and annoyed that the nursing home had, in my opinion, unnecessarily extended Norman's stay in their home needlessly but he was home now and I must think forward.

Nothing was completely new to Norman as he had seen it all during his Sunday visits. Our disabled entrance by the side of the house through the conservatory patio doors proved very easy access indeed and we parked Norman's wheelchair in the lounge next to the sofa. Kevin had cooked something for all of us to eat and we settled down together for a couple of hours. The pop-in carers were due late afternoon to help Robin to carry out personal care for Norman and put him to bed. They arrived on time and Norman was whisked away to his bedroom. Kevin and I sat on tenterhooks in the lounge. I was full of anxiety wondering how much screaming Norman was going to do. The pop-in carer was the Manager of the firm we had decided to use. He was extremely knowledgeable and showed all of the traits of an excellent carer. He and Robin seemed to be in with Norman for hours. When they finally emerged they said that Norman was in quite a state. Clearly, the day had been extremely nerve-wracking and traumatic for Norman and this had resulted in him suffering from diarrhoea. It had taken them a long time to clean him. Despite the extended personal care with new carers – not one scream, not even a murmur. We were all so pleased; I thought we had cracked it. The pop-in carer left and said he would see us in the morning.

Norman safely in bed, Robin, Kevin and I, sat in the lounge chatting getting to know each other. Robin's English was not great so this process was a little laboured. The bell that we had given Norman suddenly went off. I jumped and was so surprised because I had not known him to use his bell since early hospital days. Both Robin and I went in to see him. Norman didn't speak but we could see he was playing, mainly given away by the huge grin on his face. We spoke to him for a while and then left him and went back to the lounge. The bell went again and we returned to him. Norman continued to play like this until we told him we were going to bed and would see him in the morning. I continue to smile at this whenever I think of it because, it was the Norman I knew, his sense of humour which we no longer saw very often. Sadly though, he did not use the button again it must have been the adrenalin running through his body which gave him the motivation to be cheeky. Nevertheless that night I went to bed feeling that we had done the right thing to bring him home. The next couple of weeks were strange with us all trying to find our place and cut out a routine.

I was impressed by the pop-in Care Company insomuch as their Manager came again the next morning and for the next couple of days to help care for Norman. It surprised me though when he handed over to a trainee with no experience. Norman was the trainee's first client. The Care Company did not put too much pressure on the trainee and only gave him Norman to care for as Robin's assistant. However, he lived too far away for it to be cost effective for him to travel home and back in a few hours, so he made camp in our conservatory completing paperwork. After a couple of days, he realised that perhaps this wasn't professional but his next waiting place was in his car in our front garden. Although we never complained, it became obvious to him that camping on our doorstep was not a good idea and in another couple of days he drove down the road a mile and parked there. I felt a little sorry for him as he came across as a very caring individual but for us it was like vultures circling, waiting to pounce on Norman for his personal care. I could see that Robin was getting more and more tense regarding the assistance he was receiving. Eventually, he spoke out and asked if we could cancel the pop-in carers. Naturally I was very worried and explained to him that the nursing home had insisted on two carers for personal care. Robin explained to me that because he was 6'3" and the additional carer was much shorter, he had to position Norman's bed at the height for the additional carer. This meant that he was leaning over the bed and it was hurting his back. In addition, Robin was irritated that effectively he was training the additional carer. I could see his point of view and we had fitted a ceiling hoist on the advice of the home's Occupational Therapist as you only needed one carer with a ceiling hoist. This proved to be quite a controversial point and all throughout the time Norman was home, some agreed you only needed one carer with a ceiling hoist whilst others insisted on two carers. However, both Kevin and I were here if needed and I could fully understand Robin's concern for his own safety. So upon Robin's request we cancelled the second carer.

On the face of it this proved to be the right decision. Robin was much happier and this seemed to influence Norman. Norman was very happy to be home. Over the next few days we all got to know each other and a daily routine was established. Norman's screaming, although still being a feature, was considerably less than in the nursing home. Robin had cared for a person who was a paraplegic and was very knowledgeable and understanding regarding muscle spasms and he would use hot towels on Norman's muscles throughout the day and place his legs up in a straight position several times a day. He would also use the exercise bike that we had bought for Norman. Robin, although not experienced in using convenes, was extremely willing to learn and so this was never an issue.

He also held a British driving licence and was more than happy to take Norman out for a drive which was certainly good for him, and got Robin out of the house.

We had bought the house because of its locality only a mile from Norman's bungalow and our house which made its location very familiar to all of us. Once settled in, I asked Norman if he was happy here. To my surprise he exclaimed that it was our furniture and not his – which was true and, in fact, none of the furniture from either of our properties fitted into the house and so I said to Norman that I would go out and buy new furniture. This way it would be our (Norman's and mine) furniture – not mine or his from our old properties. His reply was yet another surprise to me which will remain in my memory banks, he said "Thank you that's kind of you." I remarked to Norman that before doing that I wanted him to revisit his bungalow to make sure that he was happy for us to sell it and for him to live at the new house. So with Robin's help, we pushed his wheelchair into the mobility vehicle and drove him a mile down the road. Observing his facial expression he was obviously pleased to be "home". It had been a long time. We had bought ramps to get Norman into the new property and we used these to get him into the bungalow. It was a challenge as it was only a two-bedroom bungalow with kitchen and lounge. The doors were narrow and on an angle. Robin did extremely well in manoeuvring Norman into the hall so that he could see the lounge, kitchen, two bedrooms as the doors all filtered off from the hall. Sadly though, the doors were too narrow to get him into the actual rooms – in fact we nearly got him stuck as it was – but Norman had seen enough to tell me that he wanted to live with us in the new house and did not want to move back. I am so pleased that we did this as we brought him back to the new property and it was clear to us all that he was going to settle in.

As I began to awaken very early one morning, shortly after Norman arrived home, I thought I must be dreaming as I could hear him shouting "Help, help," but then, startled, I realised that it *was* actually Norman shouting "Help, help." I threw some clothes on in record time and flew downstairs to him. As I entered his room I could see that he had slipped down the bed. His torso was straight, although his shoulders and head were very slightly bent left. From the waist down his legs, knees together and bent, had fallen left putting an enormous pressure on his coccyx. Tears were rolling down his face with pain. To this day, remembering this picture brings tears to my eyes. I shouted to Robin to come and help and we gently manoeuvred Norman's body into a "straight" position relieving the pressure from his lower back. Immediately his face changed as he became more comfortable. From that day forward bed positioning became a real issue to ensure that he was unable to fall left, right, or down the bed. In addition, I checked every night that the small heater was left on as I felt that maybe his body had tried to form a ball because he was cold.

Later that day, I lay in bed and put my own body into the position we found Norman feeling for myself the enormous strain and unbearable pain in my lower back.

For me, memories like this of Norman recall the evening I found him crumpled on the bathroom floor. Up until then I had always believed that life is precious and where there is life there is hope, but seeing him suffer until the day he died has often made me question that belief. I have asked myself many times "Would it have been better had Norman died that evening?" – he would have known very little about it and would not have suffered a further tortuous two years five months with very little quality of life. Now, when people tell me "So and so died suddenly", my reaction tends to be "Good for them, at least they did not suffer." I do know, however, that Norman did not want to die despite his disabilities and quality of life right up until the day he did. So, perhaps, it is a question for somebody much more intelligent than me.

The 18th of April was Norman's birthday and knowing that we were going to discharge him on the 31st March we had sent out written invitations to a party at home to celebrate his

65th birthday. Norman knew all about it and we could tell that he was quite chuffed at the thought of all the fuss he was going to receive. I was surprised and pleased to receive so many acceptances back from his friends and work colleagues, about 30 in all. We prepared lots of food and drink and discussed with Robin the best way we could deal with Norman's personal care needs in order not to embarrass anyone during the four or five hours of the party. Robin coped with this very professionally and emptied Norman's bottles without anyone noticing. Well done Robin. We were so lucky with the weather. Although it was April, we were spoilt with a day of sunshine warm enough for everyone to use the patio. At one time, I saw everyone outside whilst Norman had been left inside on his own. My heart went out to him and anyone stricken with such disabilities that they can only remain where someone puts them. I went over to him and pushed his wheelchair outside so that at least he could "people watch and listen". What was sad is that although all his friends were so sympathetic, many of them could not tolerate seeing Norman in such a way and coupled to the fact that he could not hold a conversation, just say the odd word or phrase of three or four words, not many of them visited him again. During the visit though I learnt two things about Norman, one was he knew far more of what was going on than people gave him credit for and secondly, how difficult it was for him to recall and pronounce words. During the afternoon as I approached him I could see him struggling to get my attention. As I went to him he made a great effort to say Ellen and Derek. I realised that he was asking me if we had invited them because despite everyone else being here, Norman had noticed that two of his good friends were missing. I reassured Norman that we had but clearly they could not make it, but we will ensure he visits them very shortly as they lived only a couple of miles away and this clearly pleased him. The party was a great success and we were so pleased we held it for him.

Robin could drive and so we added him to the mobility car's insurance. He was then able to take Norman to the doctors or just out for a run for fresh air. It was clear that even though it was difficult for Norman to pronounce words and hold a conversation, he still enjoyed going out and seeing people. He loved going to Duxford Air Show and, in the past, had rarely missed a show. We had taken him to Duxford from the nursing home with Dan helping us so we felt we could cope. Robin was extremely keen to go as well, so it was a treat for him. I was busy this day but Kevin, Robin and Norman went to Duxford and enjoyed a great day. Norman's friends made the usual big fuss of him and Norman's contacts meant that Robin was invited into Sally B which I had done last time we took him to Duxford. I have to say planes are far from my thing but I was so pleased I went into the Sally B. I will never forget the experience and to some degree I think it is something I can remember as sharing with Norman. What struck me in the Sally B was how on one side it was so advanced especially for its day but on the other side so basic. Walking the plank from the belly to the cockpit was quite an experience as it was so narrow and a long way down if you slipped. Closing your eyes and imagining being in that plane in the air and trying to retain your balance on this plank was quite an eye opener to what our fighter pilots went through in the world wars. Something I think we all take so much for granted. It was rewarding to take Norman out and see him enjoy himself. We felt that at least this way he had a little quality of life and decided to take him out as much as possible.

Within a couple of weeks of Norman being home, I received a telephone call from one of his friends telling me that it was the American's reunion day very soon at Horham in Suffolk the home of the Bomber Group and could we get Norman there. We knew Norman was on the committee before he fell ill and visited Suffolk at least monthly. Norman had been a regular and reliable "dishwasher" at their annual dance. Since he had fallen ill I had received many emails, get well cards, and good wishes not only from the Bomber Group in Suffolk but also from across America from those who were connected with the Bomber Group. Fred, his friend, was in his late seventies and quite active although nearly blind. Fred was also quite a chatterbox so we held the telephone to Norman's ear and let Fred chatter on for probably fifteen minutes. Norman was unable to join in the conversation but his facial expression told us that he was really enjoying hearing Fred's voice. Once Fred hung up we asked Norman if he wanted to go. His reply – the usual two words "Yes please" – but it was great to see such pleasure on his face. We promised we would take him. Plenty of organisation went into the day as it was a two-hour drive there, two hours back, plus the time spent at the reunion. Robin was extremely well organised and managed Norman's incontinence without a flaw. It was also a great day for Robin and a huge success all round. Another memorable day having discharged Norman from the neurological nursing home. It proved that: OK, Norman was now severely disabled as he had no mobility, speech difficulties, severe fatigue, incontinence and much, much more, BUT it was possible to take him out for an extremely enjoyable and rewarding day – he could still people watch, listen, and welcomingly accept a fuss being made of him. It encouraged me to take him out as much as possible and I am so pleased we did as I can now look back and say that his last months were not spent in a nursing home, they were spent out and about with his family.

When we purchased the house that we were all living in now, we had been advised that we needed a new boiler immediately, especially as it was so important to keep Norman warm. We were now a few weeks into Norman being home, so I rang and arranged for a new oil boiler to be installed replacing the old one which was housed in the utility area within kitchen cupboards. I arrived home from work on the day it was to be installed and both Robin and the engineer informed me that the kitchen cupboards would be removed, the new boiler installed, and the kitchen cupboards scrapped. I was furious and could not believe what I was hearing. Who's house was this? It was the start of coming to terms with someone living in your house and overstepping their authority. The engineer said that Robin had said it was OK to which I informed him that I was paying his company's bill, not Robin. If he was not going to reinstate the kitchen cupboards then the order would be cancelled. Needless to say, after a lot of huffing and puffing the cupboards were repositioned correctly with very little hassle. However within a couple of days of the new boiler being installed we started to get power cuts. Bizarrely, mainly at night. I slept in the room above Norman and would be woken by the alarm on his air mattress sounding. I would rush downstairs to find him laying on a completely flat mattress with no air in it at all which was very alarming because the reason he had an air mattress was due to his fragile skin and so it was imperative that the mattress stayed inflated. By now all three of us Kevin, Robin and myself were downstairs, resetting the electrical trip button and waiting for the mattress to refill before going back to bed. The same thing happened the next night and the next night – never during the day? I called and spoke to an electrician who suggested I recall out the people who had installed the oil boiler which I did. The boiler people arrived and naturally said they had done nothing wrong. We then found that a water pipe had been moved near the boiler and one of the plugs appeared wet. The electrician I had called came out and replaced the plug. Within a day or so the electrics were shorting out again, but now we could see flashing lights and the odd bang in the fuse box. Initially, I had two male adults (Kevin and Robin) running around the house trying to make out they knew what they were doing. I have to say, I was very nervous and worried and picked the telephone up to the electricians. This was now Monday and they reassured me by saying "Don't touch anything and a small crew of electricians will come out on Thursday and test the whole electrical system." I relayed this message to both Robin and Kevin and said leave everything alone. However, Kevin and I went out for a couple of hours and upon our return we were greeted by Robin saying in his broken English "I've fixed the electrics" to which I replied "Pardon?" – "I've fixed the electrics." Our faces must have been a picture. For once, due to ignorance,

I was fairly laid back. We asked Robin what he had done and he showed us that he had simply cut off the piece of wire in the plug socket behind the television that was shorting out. I didn't understand Kevin's reaction. It was now Kevin's turn to be livid saying that Robin had broken the electrical circuit. I was still laid back simply because I did not understand. However, Kevin was far from laid back he was very angry and upset which, trust me, was a rare occurrence (not like me!). I rang the electricians and told them what Robin had done. It was incredible. It reminded me of how quickly a doctor had jumped out of his chair once when I went to see him and explained that I had "red leaders" up my arm. The electricians said. "OK. We will be there first thing in the morning. We cannot get to you any earlier." Clearly, there was a huge safety issue. The electricians arrived early next morning and confirmed what Kevin had been saying. Robin had cut the electrical circuit which meant electricity was being drawn to the plug but could not return. Eventually, this would have caused a fire. We tried to explain to Robin what he had done but he remained adamant that he had sorted the problem. The electricians checked the rest of the house out and said that the lighting was sufficient but there was only one ring main for all of the plug sockets for upstairs, downstairs, the conservatory, garage and other outbuildings, which was insufficient and bordering dangerous. I explained to the electrician how disabled Norman was and how imperative it was that his room had electricity at all times. I had been told that his room was on its own circuit but the electricians confirmed that this was not accurate but it most certainly ought to be. I explained to the electricians the importance of Norman's air mattress run by electricity and how concerned I was when we lose power as not only had we had in-house problems, we had also suffered power cuts to the mains in the area. The electricians were so helpful taking on board everything I said regarding protecting Norman. They put his bedroom on a separate circuit to anything else in the house which meant any problems incurred elsewhere would not affect his room, but probably most importantly, they explained about two large batteries which we could purchase and install which would power Norman's hospital bed for 48 hours during a power cut for any reason. This idea was a huge comfort to me but, alas, it did not stop the recurring dream – of the house being on fire and I'm on my own yelling at Norman to get out of bed (which of course he couldn't) and so I grabbed him by the shoulders pulling him out of bed and letting his legs crash to the ground in a smoke-filled room – and then I woke up. This became a regular dream. The upside was that at least I must have been sleeping in order to dream.

Floorboards were taken up and the wiring for all of the sockets in the property replaced. A new mains and trips installed together with several separate circuits. Hopefully, no more problems. A few days later the power tripped out again. As promised Norman's room was not affected and he was perfectly safe with his electrical hospital bed fully functional. Needless to say, I was back on the telephone to the electricians who appeared to be just as surprised as me but, as before, they were very quick to respond and come out to investigate. It did not take them long to discover that the problem was that the electrician for the oil-fired boiler company had "nicked" a wire whilst installing the control box. Thankfully for some time after this, the electricity did not trip out but I still had my recurring dream of dragging Norman off his bed allowing him to fall to the ground in a smoke-filled room and then woke up.

It was about this time that £30 disappeared from our bedroom side table. It was the change from Duxford and Kevin and I had joked about not spending so much this time so I knew exactly how much was left. The episode also reminded me that shortly after bringing Norman home, Kevin had asked me if I had taken £10 out of his trouser pocket and we both just assumed he had been careless. Now, however, I knew for sure someone had taken £30 from my side table drawer in my bedroom. I am sure that anyone who has been burgled will understand the cold shivering sickness that waves throughout your body coupled to the feeling of being violated. Kevin and I had been married for 30 years, had chosen not to have children and so had lived our lives very privately. We knew that our decision to care for Norman at home would be a huge change to our lives but probably, ignorantly, I had not considered the feeling of not being able to relax in our own home. It was now not our home, it was a place where we slept. You could no longer leave any valuables around – although I thought we had been careful anyway. It is extremely difficult to keep things away from people either living in your house or who are regularly in and out of your house, especially when you both go out to work every day at regular times leaving the territory unguarded. I started to leave my purse in the glove compartment of my car. My car became my sanctuary but, whilst walking Jet, I realised that my car keys were hanging on the key holder in the kitchen in view of anyone who entered the house. The thought struck me that if people were willing to go upstairs when there was no reason to, then they would be quite happy to pick up by car keys whilst I'm out and look through my car. I started to carry my car keys everywhere I went which was inconvenient. One day whilst down by our garages with Jet I realised that I did not have a pocket to put my keys in but didn't want to take them back up to the house. I looked around and decided to leave them in Kevin's workshop next to the garage and went off to take Jet for his walk. Initially, on returning I forgot about the keys for a couple of hours until I wanted to use the car. Remembering what I had done I went down to Kevin's workshop to pick them up. No keys. I knew exactly where I had left them partially hidden by one of Kevin's tools. I searched and searched. No keys. Now I am thoroughly bemused. Eventually, I have no option but to give up the search and go up to the house. As I walked into the kitchen, there were my keys hanging on the key holder in the kitchen. In the short time that I had left them in the tool shed someone had been down, picked them up and placed them on the key holder. An innocent gesture I hear you all say, but I could not get my head round the question of "What were they doing in the tool shed? Why were they there? What were they doing?" The time span was so small – I felt "stalked". Was I suffering from paranoia? Discussing this with Kevin was useless (he's a man) so I discussed it with a friend. I told her what had happened and was very careful not to embellish the events as I wanted someone else's honest viewpoint. I am not sure whether I was pleased or saddened when her viewpoint was that the whole episode was very odd indeed. This now coupled to the £30 being taken meant that I was very unnerved at home. This was also made worse by seeing the flicker of a torch in our garage during the evenings which was someone riffling through our belongings which Kevin had boxed up and brought home from Norman's bungalow and our house. I finally felt it necessary to put Yale locks on our bedroom door and the office door where all of our private documents were. This gave me some reassurance that people would not be going through my private things whilst out at work or walking the dog but it was very distasteful to feel that I had to lock doors, carry the keys with me and use the glove compartment of my car to house my purse.

We also had not considered cultural differences but I do remember a couple with humour and a wry smile and, in a way, some put Robin in a child-like endearing light. Robin one day asked for the booklet for the fridge freezer which we had only just purchased and naturally I asked him why he wanted it. He said that the warning noise of the door opening annoyed him and he wanted to turn it off. I looked at him with amazement and said "No, you are not going to tamper with a brand new fridge/freezer". I came home from work another day and was unable to walk into the conservatory due to wet washing hanging from the roof struts. I immediately pulled the washing down and was greeted by Robin saying "Why are you pulling those down, they need to dry?" I'm looking at him with a blank face as I am unable to find the words to explain why. He is puzzled and I'm feeling irritated. As I walked away with the wet towels in my arm, I'm thinking "Because it is our home not a squalid bedsit or hovel". I still smile at this. All Robin wanted to do was dry the towels. It was easily solved, I asked Kevin to plumb in the tumble dryer in the garage. No more living in squalor. Whilst sitting on the sofa one day Robin came in and sat down with one of our non-stick saucepans in his hand. Clearly he was hungry and started to scoop out the contents of the saucepan with a metal spoon scraping off the non-stick surface with his spoon. I could not resist and exclaimed "We do have plates in this house you know." His reply was "It saves washing up." My reply "But we have a dishwasher. What would your Mum say?" With a smirk on his face, he said "She would tell me to go and get a plate," and then I said "And your Dad, what would he say?" Robin replied with yet another smirk and said "He would go and get another spoon and help me finish it up." This still makes me laugh; as does when Robin decided to help watering the flowers by bringing in the dirty hose from the garden, through the conservatory, across our light-coloured carpet, and out of the lounge window. "Robin, no!" I exclaimed and was greeted with his normal grin. One time Kevin told me that Robin had commented to him that I was too "posh". Possibly, this was true!

The most important thing was that Norman seemed to be as contented as he could be when taking into consideration all of his serious illnesses and Robin came across as a very caring, competent and confident, carer. We rarely saw anyone from the Company who employed him and I came to expect any meeting arranged to be cancelled but Robin had by now been with us a few weeks and things seemed to be going very well. It remained a struggle to keep the house in order as Robin seemed to want to change it into a nursing home or physiotherapy environment by leaving parts of Norman's wheelchair throughout the house, and rearranging the furniture into a waiting room. A constant battle of me explaining to Robin that the whole point of discharging Norman was for him to be in a home environment not a hospital environment. We could do little in his bedroom because of the hospital bed, ceiling hoist, wheelchair and shower chair, but the rest of the property needed to remain as a home environment. Right or wrong – you decide – I was determined to win.

The Occupational Therapist at the neurological home we had discharged Norman from had ordered Norman an extra tall shower chair due to his above average height. For the NHS this was a costly piece of equipment which had been made specifically for Norman which naturally told us that, in the OT's opinion, it was important for Norman to use it in order to keep him safe. It took a while to order and did not arrive at home until Norman had been home a few weeks. To my utter astonishment, Robin refused to use it and stored it in the garage. On asking him why, he muttered that it was not necessary. I was left questioning his decision but he had made sense when he said about hurting his back whilst placing Norman's bed at the height of a second carer but I felt that cracks were now starting to appear in Robin's care of Norman.

As mentioned earlier, Norman had been allocated a new wheelchair whilst at the nursing home which was totally unsuitable for him. Basically, it was cheap, extremely cumbersome, dangerous to push, and had insufficient cushions to cater for Norman's skin problems. By now, it was late April/May time and I had no idea who to ask or where to go but, eventually, I found out that the wheelchair centre was approximately 12 miles away.

I rang and made an appointment for an assessment. We only had to wait a few weeks for the appointment which surprised and pleased me. The day the appointment came, I'm gearing myself up for a fight as, to date, all meetings had appeared from my point of view to be bordering confrontational rather than helpful in giving Norman the best care possible. We arrived at the centre and our appointment was within a little on time. We were asked to go through to the fitting room – wheelchairs galore! The assessors were incredibly helpful. Immediately, they said without any prompting from us that the wheelchair Norman had been allocated was totally unsuitable for the same reasons as we had put forward. The requisition was completed for a tall wheelchair, with side supports, foot supports, knee supports, special cushions, and they told us it would be approximately four to six weeks. Job done. I was amazed – no fight whatsoever. We collected the wheelchair on time and left Norman's other wheelchair with them and Mark very kindly returned the borrowed wheelchair to the nursing home. Why isn't everything so professional and easy?

Mark was also very knowledgeable regarding "Comfy" chairs for the disabled and I asked for his opinion regarding one for Norman. Wheelchairs serve a very good purpose but often people do not look particularly comfortable in them. Mark explained that the "Comfy" chairs were built individually for the user; benefiting from all of the technology now used in making hospital beds to recliner chairs. Fully electric, in a variety of colours, with easy-clean fabrics. The idea of Norman sitting with us in a recliner chair in a similar colour to our furniture appealed to me as I felt, should people visit him, they will not see a huge cumbersome wheelchair which so often puts people off, they will see him sitting (hopefully) comfortably. Mark said he would forward leaflets and contact the Company that made the chairs in Wales. A few weeks later Mark and a representative arrived with a couple of sample chairs. The chairs were very adaptable; you could place them in a "resuscitation" position through to an "upright" position. Robin hoisted Norman from his wheelchair into one of the "Comfy" chairs and although Norman did not give us any verbal feedback (something we had learned to cope with), physically Kevin and I felt he looked much more comfortable than in his wheelchair. Robin surprised us all by being totally against the "Comfy" chair without offering any reasons except that it was a waste of money and not necessary. Sadly, he did not change his opinion on this, just like the "special" NHS shower chair. I decided to order a chair for Norman but was very disappointed to hear that manufacturing was six months and he would not get a chair until Christmas. It is so frustrating how long so many things take for the disabled but there did not appear to be any alternatives and so I placed the order.

Robin strongly voicing his disapproval against a "Comfy" chair was one of the many cracks that started to appear in his care of Norman. Initially it was food. Robin's eating habits were very strange. He said he was not a vegetarian but he would not eat meat. He would collect what he said were herbs whilst out walking and make green yucky drinks which he left in the fridge. More and more he controlled what and when Norman could eat. He would only allow Norman to eat rice, pasta and occasionally chicken. We tried to control this by what we bought but this was extremely difficult as we still had to buy what Robin wanted to eat. I was constantly covering up the food Robin had prepared as by now it was well into summer and living in a rural area surrounded by crops there were plenty of flies landing on Norman's food. I spoke to his employers and asked if they had given their carers any health and hygiene training especially with regard to the preparation of food but this appeared to fall on very deaf ears. All I could do was keep my eyes open. Kevin one day said to Robin that Norman liked to eat meat and Robin told Kevin that he was Norman's carer, not Kevin, and Norman would eat what Robin decided. Understandably, this angered Kevin. Again we tried to control this by telling Robin that we would cook Norman's main meal and he would eat with us, but Robin became more and more crafty and would feed Norman earlier and earlier and when we came home, we found Norman already in bed. One day, Kevin and I decided to take the direct route and told Robin that there was a prepared chicken meal in the freezer for Norman to eat. Reluctantly he agreed to give this to Norman. Kevin and I went out and as we were driving down the road, Kevin suddenly said is Robin cooking that chicken now? We rushed back to check and yes Robin was cooking the chicken from frozen despite the warning on the packet to ensure that the meal is fully defrosted first. We snatched the meal away from Robin. More and more doubt was setting in regarding trusting Robin to prepare Norman's food. I was also very worried as to whether or not he was feeding the herbs (weeds) he was collecting whilst out walking to Norman. Sadly, Norman was always the only one that suffered and Robin's diet was causing him to suffer from diarrhoea and constipation which was then controlled by giving him Movicol. Once we were able to gain control of Norman's diet these problems improved.

I had made several enquiries, once I knew we were discharging Norman, to various physios and had discovered that Norman required a specially-training neuro physio. I was surprised to find one practicing in our town just six miles away from the house. I contacted them and they were very happy to come out and assess Norman. It was a huge relief to me that they were willing to make house visits as several physios will only treat their clients at their own premises.

A visit was arranged and the physio visited Norman. He complimented Robin's positioning of Norman's legs in that Robin regularly put his legs up on a chair to straighten them. The physio also gave us flexion exercises to do and Robin showed him the bike we had bought (which was exactly the same as the nursing home used) to exercise Norman's legs. For me, it was a comforting visit reassuring our care of Norman and we agreed that he would visit us at home once a month. To my surprise, Robin expressed his annoyance that I had called in a physio as he considered it unnecessary. He added that the physio did not know any more than he did and that he was perfectly capable in doing the necessary exercises which, to be fair, he was, but his attitude was less than favourable. A few days later, I came home from work to be greeted by a chilling scream from Norman. As I walked into the lounge, Robin was standing in front of Norman's wheelchair and holding both of his hands at his own waist height. Norman's facial expression was one of sheer terror. His face was distorted with fear and tears welling up in his eyes. "Robin, what are you doing?" I shouted. He replied in his broken English "Helping Norman to walk." "But Robin, Norman is petrified – look what you are doing to him – you know he cannot walk – stop it." Robin let go of Norman's hands and stepped back, Norman stopped screaming but looked terrified and to me looked like he was physically shaking. With some sort of order re-established and Norman settling down; I grabbed my mobile phone and rang the neuro physio. He always proved to be a great comfort to me as he would discuss my concerns and would invariably take my call. With a very shaky voice I explained to the physio what I had just witnessed. I have always believed in not exaggerating and so, yet again, I was very careful to just relay to him what I had seen and asked his advice as to whether or not I was overreacting. I think the physio too, was shell-shocked, at what I was telling him as I had to repeat it a couple of times. Clearly, he too did not understand the thinking behind Robin's actions but he assured me that this was totally unacceptable. In many ways, I think Robin was trying to motivate Norman and simply did not see the harm he was doing or could do.

I still smirk, when remembering another day. I went down to the garage to see a hose pipe attached to Norman's right hand and pointing at my car with the water running. Robin was kindly washing my car using washing up liquid. This time there was a smile on Norman's face which was good to see. Yet another day I caught Robin wrapping Jet's lead round Norman's right hand. Jet was very strong and could have caused enormous damage to Norman but Robin could not see this.

The summer was marching on now and we had been exceptionally lucky with the weather. Robin had been with us for best part of three months and had another month to go. He was clearly tired and needed a holiday and this began to show in his care of Norman. Kevin was becoming more and more agitated with Robin's insistence that he "was in charge of Norman," and more and more nagging doubts were entering my thoughts . I was now very concerned regarding Norman's safety with a view to the food Robin insisted on feeding him and the fact that I had witnessed Robin tying Jet's lead to his wrist. For me, the wheelchair incident when Robin was trying to get Norman to stand was very difficult to understand or forgive. I was now also, concerned regarding all of our safety following Robin cutting the electrical plug circuit. Once nagging doubt sets in, it is very difficult to eliminate it. Maybe if I had not been so worried regarding Norman's care/safety, I may have been able to overlook the other issues. So after very careful consideration I decided to let the Care Company know my feelings and notified them that it was probably best if Robin did not return after his holiday. I still wonder even today if it was the right decision but I no longer could trust him with Norman or the house and, at this moment in time, I was confident that the Care Company had a pool of qualified carers and would be able to replace Robin easily.

Reflecting on the summer, I believe we all had an enjoyable time, including Norman. We had taken Robin to several places, including twice to Duxford Air Show, Suffolk Bomber Group, Colchester Zoo, Colchester Castle, Heavy Horse and Veteran Motor show, Maldon sea side and much more. We had been out nearly every week end and I do not regret one moment of it. Norman's last summer was the best we were able to give him.

It is now nearing the end of July and Robin cannot wait for his holiday and who can blame him? It is the procedure for the carer who is taking over to spend a day with the carer going off on holiday. So the day before Robin was due to fly out our new carer arrived. He slept in Robin's room and we made a bed up for Robin in another room. At 7.30 a.m. the next day I was informed by the new carer that he was not going to stay as he would not be able to cope with Norman. The new carer had had a good night's sleep, shower, and breakfast, left his towels folded outside the bathroom, and was now on his way back home. Needless to say, Robin was panicked. He wanted/needed his holiday. The telephone was hot with calls to/from the Care Company.

Whilst waiting for their call back I walked into the kitchen to see Robin curled up under the sink and I asked "What are you doing?". He replied in his broken English, "I need to know where the water is coming from." "Why?" I asked. "Because I need to know." "But Robin I need to know why you need to know?" I exclaimed. "I need to know what is killing me," he replied. To this day, whenever I have any doubts regarding Robin, I remember this last encounter. I think his problem was that our kettle furred up very easily due to having hard water, and it was the scaling that was worrying him, but it is only a guess.

Within half an hour of Robin leaving to catch his plane, the new carer arrived. The handover from Robin to the new carer Mathew was less than half an hour and Robin was gone.

Mathew

The Manager of the Care Company told me that Mathew did not tick all of the boxes she and I discussed at the nursing home prior to Norman's discharge but, at this moment in time, she did not have an alternative. She also told me that she was not sure of Mathew's suitability and would continue to look for a more suitable carer.

Possibly, the problems with Mathew were, firstly cultural because he was African and, secondly, the fact that he did not drive. Not being able to drive had many knock-on problems. The house was approximately six miles from the local town and so you needed a car to travel anywhere. The location was in a rural part of the country and although we have half a dozen neighbours, there is very little to do unless you like walking. It is a picturesque part of the world with many paths to walk. Mathew not being able to drive also meant that he was unable to take Norman out and about whilst both Kevin and I were at work. Also, it was now down to either Kevin or myself to collect Norman's medication and to drive him to any medical or any other appointment. The extra chores did not phase either Kevin or myself as we were perfectly happy to drive Norman wherever he needed to go, but it did mean that he spent more time indoors than perhaps we would have liked. However

Mathew was here with us now and we needed to make the most of the situation.

Initially, I felt compassion for Mathew as he had been kind enough to come to us with very short notice, little preparation and next to no handover from Robin. Robin had left Norman in his wheelchair with us in the lounge and Mathew also sat with us. We all enjoyed an evening meal and once finished, the evening started to march on until late for Norman to be transferred to bed and I felt the need to ask Mathew if he was going to put him to bed. His face glazed over and there was obviously a problem. It transpired that Mathew had no idea as to how to use the ceiling hoist or sling. This was our first very important lesson on the lack of training of carers and it also highlighted that to some degree we had taken Robin for granted as we had nothing to compare him against. It was now quite late and Norman needed to go to bed. I logged on to the internet to download instructions on using the slings and hoist for Mathew to read whilst Kevin became the guinea pig in the hoist instructing Mathew how to put the sling on and use the hoist. After approximately an hour of Kevin being hoisted in and out of bed by Mathew; Mathew swatting up on the paperwork I had downloaded, we all felt it was safe to hoist Norman into bed. Mathew also needed training on the use of convenes and he was not particularly happy that he did not have another carer to help. To be fair to Mathew he had been expecting another carer on-site to help him. Robin had never told his Company that he was working alone and although his Manager had made appointments to visit us, she had cancelled every one and so had not actually visited to supervise Robin or talk to us.

Mathew learnt how to use the ceiling hoist, convenes, and seemed to become quite competent and confident in looking after Norman, relatively quickly. Initially, he was very talkative and seemed to like his room and the location of the house. Mathew was far more open to Norman's food requirements and it was not long before we found ourselves in the routine of eating as a family. Norman did need support whilst eating but this was not a problem. We explained to Mathew about the shower chair which had been ordered specifically for Norman by the NHS which was sitting in the garage as Robin had refused to use it and he went to have a look. From that day forward the extra tall shower chair was used and every carer found it more than suitable, so we still have no idea why Robin was so against it.

Robin had commented before his holiday that it was becoming more and more difficult to persuade Norman to drink and this became very evident with someone else caring for him but, initially, Mathew seemed to have this under control.

As the days past, Mathew seemed to find a routine. It was difficult for him as Norman did not seem to take to him and started to scream during personal care again. I tried to help the best I could by going to Norman's room and sitting by the door to comfort him. Mathew said several times that this helped him as Norman did not scream anywhere as much or as loud if I was close by. This did lead, however, to Mathew believing that I should be the one carrying out personal care; he did not seem to accept that I wanted to keep some form of dignity for Norman and remain "a sister". During the earlier days Norman and I had agreed that he did not want me to carry out personal care and I have to admit, I did not want to be a "hands-on" carer. Mathew would leave the door open throughout personal care which I felt compromised Norman's dignity to a degree but I did not consider it serious enough to comment.

I notified the neuro physio that we had a new carer and asked if he could come out and show Mathew what to do regarding the exercises Norman needed and putting his legs up and down in order to straighten his knees.

During his time off, Mathew asked me if he could accompany me whilst I took Jet for his walk so that he could get some fresh air away from the house whilst Kevin stayed at home to look after Norman. Naturally, I was only too happy to show him the area as I appreciated he needed a break from the house. He clearly enjoyed the countryside and the number of footpaths nearby and, at one point, he commented that it reminded him of home.

Whilst out walking Mathew was constantly saying that he was here now to care for Norman and I no longer needed to worry about him. He said over and over that he was a good carer but, if he did something not to our liking, then to speak up and tell him as he wanted to do exactly as we wanted. Many times as I left for work in the morning, Mathew would compliment me saying how nice and smart I looked going off to work which I thanked him for but took no notice.

One day when arriving home after work (about 4 p.m.) both Kevin and Mathew "pounced" on me telling me that the electrics were not working on Norman's hospital bed. Kevin said he had checked the attachments underneath the bed which had come apart before but they were OK. Naturally, I asked if either of them had contacted the maintenance company for the bed who were on a 24-hour call out. Both Kevin and Mathew said that they had both rung independently but the maintenance company would not come out for 48 hours. I immediately picked the telephone up and, as I did so, both Kevin and Mathew said that I was wasting my time. I spoke to the receptionist of the maintenance company reiterating that both my husband and the carer for my brother, who was seriously disabled and needed the electrics to be working on his hospital bed, had called earlier asking for a maintenance call. Politely, she informed me that they would be out in 48 hours. I explained again and she said "She knew how I felt but . . ." to which I replied "No, you do not know how I feel unless you have a family member in a hospital bed with failed electrics. No electrics means that we cannot raise Norman into a sitting position in order to give him a drink or something to eat. Norman is totally reliant on the bed's electrics to move." She replied "They could not come out for 48 hours." I reminded her that they advertised a 24-hour service to which she answered that was a telephone call service only, not maintenance. I asked to speak to her Manager and she said he would say the same. After thirty minutes or more she realised that I was not going to put the telephone down until someone came out as I was not prepared to leave Norman lying flat on his back for 48 hours, unable to give him a drink or food, and she transferred me to her Manager. He gave me the same story and I reiterated the urgency. Finally, he also realised that I was not going to put the telephone down and he asked me to hold. After a few moments, he returned to the telephone and said that someone would be with me at approximately 6 p.m. as they would call in on their way home. I thanked him profusely and awaited the engineer. The engineer duly arrived at 6 p.m. with two replacement handsets – that is all that was wrong. The engineer replaced the handset (took one minute) and gave us a spare telling us to keep it as the problem is invariably the handset. I thanked him and off he went home but it was another lesson on how vulnerable severely disabled people, like Norman, are when out of a hospital environment and how tough and dogmatic you have to be in order to obtain what they need. Both Kevin and Mathew were dumfounded and I just said I was not coming off the telephone until they came out.

Mathew was with us for approximately four weeks and then left for a week's holiday. Upon his return he notified us that he had asked to be replaced as he had decided to retire and return to Africa. Both Kevin and I understood and supported his decision and wished him well.

Unfortunately, however, the Care Company did not have another suitable carer to replace Mathew and told him that he would have to stay until they found a replacement. With the benefit of hindsight, Mathew changed from this point forward. He no longer stayed downstairs with us but retreated to his bedroom. He would sit on the sofa in the mornings biting his nails telling me that he dreaded going in to carry out Norman's personal care. He complained about the carer who had looked after Norman for the week he was away, showing me photographs of dirt under Norman's fingernails. Mathew constantly told me that he was a good carer. To be honest, I probably did not realise how serious the situation was becoming, as I was expecting him to be transferred. Kevin also did not tell me that Mathew was now repeatedly complaining to him about me saying that I should be at home caring for Norman (I was out working as I was the main breadwinner nowadays as Kevin had semi-retired) and telling Kevin that he (Kevin) was the man of the house. Mathew had also told me several times that Kevin was the "man of the house". He now went to Kevin rather than me if he needed to ask anything. This made me smile as, in fact, the house belonged to Norman so actually Norman was "the man of the house". I later learnt that Mathew had also complained to the Manager of the Care Company about Kevin not being "man of the house" which was yet another enormous invasion of our privacy and example of cultural differences.

One day, Norman was not particularly well (probably due to another urine infection) and I asked the doctor to call. I left work early to meet the doctor at home and, on arrival, I asked where Mathew was. Mathew had put the lead on Jet and gone out for a walk even though he knew he would miss the doctor – he had asked Kevin if it was OK and Kevin had said yes (you are absolutely right, I wasn't too happy with Kevin either). Needless to say when the doctor arrived and wanted to clarify a few points with Norman's carer, I was embarrassed to report that Mathew was out walking the dog.

Kevin and I became increasingly worried as we were no longer seeing Norman's legs up on a chair and his screaming was escalating. The physio was still only visiting monthly and I rang and asked for an urgent visit. The physio confirmed that there was a significant decline in Norman's mobility and possibly the formation of contractures and suggested writing to his doctor with a view to "botox" treatment. The doctor, in turn, suggested asking the NHS Occupational Therapist for Bed Positioning to visit and advise and, naturally, I was more than willing for the doctor to arrange a meeting with them. The physio also suggested purchasing a positioning T-roll which could be placed between Norman's knees in bed which would help in keeping his knees apart and his hips in alignment together with a knee brace which may help to straighten his left knee. Both were subsequently purchased. The physio also confirmed that Norman's decline was probably not helped by Mathew not carrying out the recommended exercises despite my calling out the physio immediately that Mathew had arrived, to ensure that he was fully aware and trained regarding Norman's physio care needs.

I instantly realised that part of the problem was that Mathew was employed by the Care Company and would only do what they instructed him to do. I rang the Manager of the Care Company and the physio and asked if they would both visit the house to discuss the need and importance of these exercises. Both agreed and a date was arranged for the coming Friday. However, the Thursday before the meeting, whilst we were all sitting eating our evening meal, Mathew got up to fill the dishwasher. I looked over and saw that Norman was struggling to eat his meal and so naturally went over to him to help. Kevin and Mathew were in the kitchen. When Norman had finished, I took his plate into the kitchen. As I walked into the room, Mathew flew at me shouting something like "I don't play games. If you want to do my job, then I can leave now. I don't have to stay here and take this …" Kevin's jaw was on the floor. Confused and bewildered, I replied "Mathew I'm helping to feed my brother because you are busy, if you would like to do it then please carry on." Mathew flew at me again shouting that he was a good carer and then stormed upstairs into his bedroom. Nothing more was said that night and Mathew looked after Norman regarding putting him to bed and his personal care etc., but he stayed well away from Kevin and I.

Early the next morning I rang the Manager of the Care Company and told her what had happened and she tried to reassure me by saying that Mathew was due to be replaced by another carer within a week or two. I expressed my concern regarding his threatening behaviour towards me and his outburst saying that he was going to walk out. The Manager arrived later that day in time for our meeting with the physio which went very well. Mathew was present but we all recognised that really the purpose of this meeting was for the Care Company to include in their care package the exercises that Norman needed. After the meeting, the Manager assured me that after a long conversation with Mathew she was confident that he would not walk out and would carry out the exercises that Norman needed whilst he was here. She realised that this was simply a case of lifting Norman's arms or legs and flexing the joints before hoisting and also lifting the legs off the wheelchair onto a chair so that his knees were straightened for a couple of hours.

The next day, Saturday, I said good morning to Norman and Mathew appeared to be OK. I left the house for a couple of hours and upon return asked Mathew if we could put Norman's legs up as agreed yesterday. Mathew stormed in from the kitchen saying that he was preparing a drink for Norman and shouting at me. He was then sarcastic – "So, you want his legs up?" I replied, "Yes please." Mathew then asked "How?" and I replied, "As suggested and agreed with the physio yesterday please." I managed to get Norman's left leg up, when Mathew jumped back from me shouting "You don't scare me; you don't tell me what to do…" I have to say I did say quietly and calmly "For goodness sake Mathew grow up," at which point he stormed upstairs to his bedroom, threw his clothes into a suitcase and came back downstairs shouting aggressively "You had better call the office - I'm leaving" and stormed out of the house to sit on the front garden wall. By now Norman was extremely agitated and upset. Despite all of his disabilities he knew Mathew was threatening me with his behaviour and Norman, my big brov, would have always protected me in the past and now, of course, he couldn't. I reassured Norman and put his left leg down so that he was comfortable and stayed with him until he settled as I saw tears whelming up in his eyes. Within half an hour Kevin came home, driving past Mathew sitting on the front wall with his suitcase by his side. Kevin came straight into the lounge where I was sitting with Norman and asked what was going on. I told him what had happened and understandably he was not surprised having witnessed Mathew's outburst less than 48 hours ago for absolutely no reason. I rang the Care Company who, at this point, would not take my call as they wanted to talk to Mathew first to obtain his side of the story. Eventually, the telephone rang and it was the Care Company. They asked what had happened and I started to tell them over the telephone but burst into tears. The Care Company realised that they needed to find a replacement carer immediately and rang off to start looking. It was clear that they had told Mathew that he was not allowed to leave the location until a replacement carer had been found and so he remained sitting on the wall of our front garden.

An hour or so later, the Care Company rang and said that they had found someone willing to come out providing it was a permanent position. I was honest with the Care Company saying that I could not guarantee that it was a permanent position. It was clear to them from my voice that I was extremely upset and they told me someone would be with me as soon as possible. Mathew sat on the front wall for the next four to five hours until someone arrived. She came into the house and asked if Mathew could come back into the property in order to handover to her. Naturally I said of course that was no problem. My only priority was the care of Norman. Another short handover took place and Mathew was gone and, until this day, I have no idea what I did to Mathew as my only interference with his care of Norman was to sit close to Norman when his screaming was escalating. It will always remain a mystery and can only be explained by cultural differences – I'm not "the little woman" I should be in Mathew's eyes.

Zara

As I showed Zara to her bedroom, Jet was at my heel which was normal as he tended to be my shadow. Zara surprised me by exclaiming – "He doesn't come in the house does he?" I replied

111

"Of course he does, he lives here." Exasperated Zara exclaimed – "But he won't come upstairs and into my bedroom will he?" I tried to reassure her that Jet was an adorable dog and, generally speaking, he did not go upstairs but suggested that she kept her bedroom door closed as a precaution.

Speaking to Zara, I soon realised that she was not experienced enough to cope with Norman. She had had only two weeks' training on how to care for people. She had no idea how to use a hoist, hospital bed, slings, slip sheets, convenes, skin issues, etc. In fact, we might as well have just gone out and pulled someone off the streets. I was extremely anxious.

Luckily, Denise, a friend of mine who was now a police officer, had trained as a carer. Norman knew her and responded well to her. I rang her and through my tears told her what had happened. She immediately said she would help as much as possible and its friends like her who are so precious. I went to collect her and when we arrived back at the house we saw Jet outside in the garden which was extremely unusual as he stayed in the house enjoying his home comforts. Denise loved animals, especially Jet, and asked what he was doing outside and I replied that I had no idea. As we approached the back door to the house, we saw Jet's bed neatly folded and placed by the backdoor. Clearly, Zara had put him out into the back garden as soon as I had left the house.

Denise came into the house and spoke to Norman. She worked shift work and said that she would be here to care for Norman whenever she could but still had to go to work. Kevin's brother had also trained as a carer and was now retired. So we picked the telephone up and by 5 p.m. we had arranged for Norman to be cared for between Denise, Robert and Zara, with Kevin and I, helping as much as possible in between our own work commitments – which is why we had chosen to have a live-in carer in the first place.

Norman responded well to both Denise and Robert caring for him as they were familiar to him and English with a sense of humour he understood and recognised. Zara displayed an exceptional attitude towards learning and showed a natural compassion towards the disabled. Denise and Robert drew up a rota and trained her for the next two weeks. Every morning when I woke up for the next two weeks, I would come downstairs to find her sitting in the conservatory. Immediately, she put pressure on me to give her a permanent position. However, by now I was showing signs of the pressure of looking after Norman myself and bursting into tears throughout the day at any time, especially when she put pressure on me regarding a permanent position. I think she would have made an excellent carer as she was so willing to learn and wanted to do a good job. I tried to explain to her that over the past months I had realised that the Care Company did not have access to a pool of qualified carers that they had led me to believe they had and I needed continuity of qualified care for Norman. I remembered the "joy" I had clocked when the Manager of the Care Company had told me excitedly that they had found a suitable carer and I now understood why she was so pleased. I could not risk Norman's safety with untrained carers. Zara was intelligent and could see just how upset I was, bordering on my own depression caused by the situation. Zara was also very angry with the Care Company as she felt that they had been far from honest with her. At this point, it seemed that my only choice was to contact a local Pop-In Care Company and make alternative arrangements with them as I felt sure they would have sufficient qualified carers on their books to provide me with the continuity of care that I needed for Norman. Both Kevin and I realised that it was almost impossible to live with carers from abroad due to the cultural differences. Something which had never crossed our minds at the start of this process and the bizarre thing is that neither Kevin nor I dictated to the carers, it was the carers employed by us who were inflicting their ways upon us. At this point, I also realised the extent of the lack of training these carers received on how to care for people as ill as Norman.

Chapter 5
Pop-In Carers

My enquiries led me to a local company who had a good reputation and so I rang and gave them a brief outline of my predicament. They were extremely understanding and supportive over the telephone and we made an appointment to meet and discuss the care of Norman. It was clear to me that Denise and Robert could only look after Norman in the short-term and although Zara was furthering her training daily with them, it was obvious I would be in the same situation when she left so I needed to get something organised as soon as possible.

Taking yet another day off work (my boss's understanding was faultless), I met the Manager of the Pop-In Care Company and spent several hours explaining Norman's illnesses and extensive care needs. Most of the time, tears were rolling down my face as I seemed to be crying for no reason throughout the day at this point. The Manager surprised me by saying "You are no ogre; you just haven't received the right amount of support". We parted, having arranged for a carer to look after Norman from 8 a.m. to 5 p.m. whilst both Kevin and I were at work, and for a second carer to come in four times a day to carry out personal care. Although still tearful, I felt happier especially as I was able to tell Denise and Robert that the new company would start within a week or so.

The first day came for the new Care Company to start and I opened the door to the carer. Immediately, she asked if I could give her some background as to why she was there and what was expected from her. Yet again, my face was a picture. I said that I had spent several hours explaining Norman's needs to her Manager so surely you have been briefed? She said she had been told nothing. I rang the Care Company who, in turn, asked to speak to the carer. I was late for work that day as I sat and briefed the carer regarding Norman's needs. This became a regular habit when a new carer arrived. Within five days, I realised what a catastrophic mistake I had made and started to consider my alternatives.

The carer who came from 8 a.m. to 5 p.m. basically "house sat". She was very willing to do the ironing or hovering but that was not part of the arrangement. The arrangement was to care for Norman. She would not do anything for Norman on her own. The second carer that came in was very much in Norman's face. Her heart was in the right place as she was just trying to "connect" with him, but she was far too overbearing for Norman. She repeatedly said to him (six inches away from his face) - "My name is Michaela, Michaela; my name is Michaela, Michaela, what is my name?" I was not at all surprised when Norman did not answer and so she repeated "My name is Michaela, Michaela, what is my name?"

Eventually, Norman answered "Margaret" and, immediately, I had to walk away in an attempt to hide the smile on my face which was bursting into a laugh. Well done Norman! To this day, I like to think that replying Margaret instead of Michaela was his sense of humour. It certainly would have been prior to him falling ill!

It is now November and the local pub has held an annual firework display for the past few years. Knowing that Norman has attended this event before I asked him if he wanted to go and he eagerly replied "Yes". Four of us parcelled him in to our mobility car and set off looking forward to a great evening. As we arrive, several people were queuing to enter which was quite normal and we chatted whilst waiting our turn. Once in the two acre field we parked Norman's wheelchair at the back away from the crowds remembering our experience of

Norman and crowds at Duxford. We were all standing around Norman chatting and looking forward to the display as in the past it has been extremely good. As expected the display started with two extremely large "bangs" followed closely by several large rockets and we are all staring into the sky watching the fireworks. Suddenly, I heard a whimper and as I look down at Norman I saw that he was shaking, his face crumpled, and tears were rolling down his face – a reaction from him that I had not considered or expected. Was he scared? Was he crying because he was remembering happier times in years gone by? I had no idea. We tried to console him the best we could but he continued to cry. Quickly, we pushed the wheelchair back to where the car was parked and loaded him. Once in the mobility car he settled and the tears disappeared. It was yet another example of just how fragile Norman had become and I would have to give greater consideration to where we took him in the future.

Each evening within a short time of the pop-in carers' arrival, Kevin and I were very bemused walking around the house trying to find what was the source of the burning we could smell. It took a while, but one night as I went into the porch I saw smoke coming from the porch lights and as I looked up to the lights I could see that the ceiling was burning around every light. Can you believe it – more electrical problems. Up until now it had been daylight and we had not needed to put the porch lights on. I certainly did not like seeing smoke coming from the ceiling and rang my trusty electricians the next morning. As I had come to expect they arrived and replaced the lights professionally and without fuss but my recurring dream of dragging Norman out of a burning house returned for a few nights.

I was beginning to realise that the only way I was going to get Norman cared for to the standard he deserved was to employ carers direct under PAYE and so I started to make enquiries as to how I was going to achieve this. Firstly, I needed to advertise for carers and secondly, I needed to register Norman as an employer and set up a payroll.

Meanwhile, daily, Norman's screaming began to escalate. It was clear that he was far from happy with the care he was receiving. After a couple of weeks, he looked, dirty, unshaven and extremely unhappy. We started to look through the daily care notes and found that he had not received a shower for at least ten days. I rang the Care Company and made arrangements for them to visit. A carer arrived that day who I had not seen before. I went into Norman's room to see her giving him medication from the drawers. I asked what she was doing and why was she not giving him the medication from the dosette box? She had referred to the medication list in the file. I said to her to look at the date and that Norman's medication had been in a dosette box since we discharged him home. The colour drained out of her face. I knew what medication was in the drawer and also knew that none of it was dangerous. I felt that I was in the wrong to have left the medication in the drawer but it had not crossed my mind that carers would ignore the dosette box which was fully in view. The carer looked white and shaken and I could not leave her in that state for any longer than a few minutes. I said to her: "Let's go through together what you have given him" and luckily, as I say, there was nothing of any danger but I did feel it was a lesson that she will never forget.

The Manager arrived and I led her in to see Norman. You could see from her face that she was not impressed and to be fair to her she said that she would not wish a family member of hers to be neglected in such a way. She also said that she and the carer would give Norman a shower immediately.

After the shower, the Manager sat down with me to discuss the way forward and her recommendation was to increase the number and frequency of carers attending increasing the cost significantly. I decided to agree to this as I had already found a directly-employed carer but had to wait for him to work his notice. I was hoping this would be three or four weeks but it turned out to be five weeks. It was a very long and stressful five weeks, especially for Norman.

Norman needed to have convenes fitted but due to its very personal nature the carers working for the Care Company refused to use them and would only fit pads – often double padding which I was informed later by the incontinent team can cause skin breakdown. Wanting to make sure my facts were straight I rang and spoke to the doctor who confirmed that, due to Norman's skin problems, convenes needed to be used as much as possible and he would organise the incontinence team to visit. I contacted the Care Company and informed them of this and asked that they visit at the same time as the incontinence nurse. The incontinence nurse visited and found that there were additional problems insomuch as Norman was suffering from penis retraction that made fitting the convenes quite tricky but because of his skin breakdown on his private parts every effort must be made to use the convenes. The incontinence nurse would, however, order different pads but again emphasised that convenes must be used as much as possible. Despite being told by the professionals, the carers continued to fight the use of convenes using pads as a preference. The carers would also clean Norman's private parts using baby wipes only and not water. During one of my conversations with the pop-in carers, one of them said to me "But you have to realise how little these carers are being paid" to which I replied "No, you have to realise the enormous amount or money Norman is paying for inadequate care."

We saw a significant difference in Norman each week the pop-in carers continued to care for him. It was clear that Norman could not cope with this type of care. Possibly, it reminded him of the nursing home. Within two to three weeks, his screaming had escalated to throughout the day and not just during personal care. I would stay with him when I was not at work which did help, but one day as I arrived home from work and walked into the lounge Norman told me to "F… Off". The NHS nurses, who had visited Norman approximately twice a week since his discharge, also recognised how unhappy he was and reported this on their daily logs and to their Manager and his doctor. By now, I had arranged for two direct-carers to start and was counting the days.

One night as Norman sat in his Comfy Chair awaiting the pop-in carers to arrive he started to scream and scream. Kevin walked out and I burst into tears. Norman stopped screaming and started to repeat "Sorry, sorry." I jumped up and went over to him and hugged him and said "Norman I'm doing the best I can and I'm sorry if it is not good enough." Norman replied "It is." The pop-in carers arrived and picked up on the atmosphere but had no idea why.

It was now December and Christmas was not far away. My new directly-employed carer Peter said that he would cover Christmas because in his experience people were often let down over Christmas by pop-in carers. Peter had also been out of caring for a couple of years and we agreed to keep the pop-in carers coming in for a few days so that he could adjust easily.

Chapter 6
Peter and Cassandra

Peter and Cassandra became directly-employed carers for Norman at the end of December. They were both a breath of fresh air. I was now able to personally compile Norman's care plan and encompass all of his care needs and know that it would be complied with without fuss or cultural differences.

They both worked a split shift. Peter worked from 8.30 a.m. to 5 p.m. and from 8 p.m. to 9 p.m. Monday to Friday, and Cassandra worked the same hours Saturday and Sunday. Naturally, I was very open if they wanted to change days at any time for a day off. We also had Robert and Denise as emergency carers and obviously Kevin and I were available when not working. I did not know at the time and to be honest found out a little late that the NHS Provide Nurses would also provide emergency cover if needed and it would have been very useful to have known this earlier. So often throughout this process I have found out about services that are available to disabled people too late and have often wondered why nobody tells you sooner. It is a mystery.

Peter and Cassandra worked extremely well together covering Norman's needs. The neuro physio had been coming out weekly to Norman since our problems with Mathew and I felt confident now to ask him out to show Peter and Cassandra the exercises he needed. No longer did I have a fight on my hands to ensure these exercises were carried out. No longer did

I have a fight on my hands to ensure that convenes were used as much as possible and no longer did I have to worry about the food Norman was being fed or regarding the care of his fragile skin. The difference in the skill and training of these two carers coupled to no cultural differences improved the quality and reduced the stress in all of our lives enormously – especially for Norman. They both drove and Peter, in particular, was happy to take Norman out during the week for a drive and to collect his medication etc.

It was now January and our appointments which I had requested during June (seven months earlier) were nearly upon us. The first appointment I had requested was to see a consultant for Norman's rheumatoid arthritis as he had not seen one for at least two to three years. We all went, Peter, Kevin Norman and myself. It proved to be extremely helpful to both Peter and I and it was a shame that we had had to wait for over seven months for the appointment. The consultant advised us that although Norman's rheumatoid arthritis was dormant at the moment, he would still be suffering enormous pain when his joints were moved, especially after being set in one position for some time – could this be part of the reason(s) for Norman's screaming. The consultant told us that painkillers such as paracetamol (used by the nursing home) were not effective and advised us to experiment with co-codamol – obviously keeping within the advised dosages. This advice proved to be extremely useful. We experimented as much as possible and found that Norman benefited from being given two co-codamol tablets 30 minutes before being hoisted. It saddens me that the nursing home seemed to be unaware of the painful symptoms of rheumatoid arthritis, let alone general neuropathy and, possibly due to ignorance had used paracetamol which did not help Norman at all, instead of co-codamol and we, in turn, had not been made aware of this until now.

The second appointment I requested was to see a neurologist as I had been told that Norman was suffering from a brain disease and I felt that the word "disease" meant that his condition was progressive. The neurologist described him as being "mute" and suggested that it may be of benefit to contact our local palliative care hospice. It was clear that the neurologist did not believe that this was registering with Norman but Peter, Kevin and I, knew it was. The neurologist also suggested that it would be beneficial for Norman to have another scan and told us that he would make an appointment with our local hospital.

On arriving back home, I knew Norman had heard and understood "palliative care". I asked Peter what he thought and he said that he felt that Norman was particularly quiet and reserved. Norman was extremely intelligent and I knew that it was going to be difficult to persuade him that he was not dying. However, we had to try. All three of us spoke to him separately and Kevin then took a dictionary into him which gave a definition of palliative care as being the control of pain. Norman seemed to cheer up slightly although to this day I am unconvinced. Right or wrong, I felt irritated by the neurologist for putting Norman through this added, unnecessary, distress. He did not have to mention "palliative care" in front of Norman. The day came for his scan and Peter and I set off to the hospital for our appointment. Needless to say, we were kept waiting for some time and eventually someone came out to us and suggested we make our way down the stairs to the front of the building, where the portacabin was located. I asked if the portacabin housed or had access to a hoist. The person replied "No". I explained Norman's condition and she stated that we should have noted that on the application for the appointment – the trouble was; we did not make the appointment – the doctor did. However, she said to wait here and she would be back. She came back and told us to make our way to another part of the hospital which did have a hoist over the scanner. Once there, we sat and waited and waited and waited, as per normal. I was getting very concerned for Norman as by now he had been sitting in his wheelchair too many hours for his various conditions and sensitive skin, but there was nothing I could do. Eventually, someone came out and invited us in – all other patients had been seen and we had been left to last – it continues to amaze me how so little thought or understanding is given to the seriously ill/disabled – don't they know that there is often a time limit to how long an individual can sit in a wheelchair? So often throughout this journey people have quoted to me "duty of care; best interests", but rarely have I seen these phrases adhered to. Anyway, it was down to Peter to use their hoist and place Norman on the scanner as they did not have a skilled member of staff available. Naturally, Peter was more than happy to do this. Norman became quite distressed and agitated but we were able to calm him especially as Peter was in charge and Norman trusted him, so it actually worked in our favour that they did not have a skilled member of staff available. Several hours late; we were on our way home and I could not help but think how inconsiderate and lacking in compassion it was to leave such a seriously disabled individual to last. The scan confirmed that there had been further episodes (mini strokes) within Norman's brain which helped us to understand his decline.

A few months ago, I had agreed for the doctor to ask the NHS Occupational Therapist for Bed Positioning to visit and today was the day. Promptly, two people arrived and after the normal "niceties" started to explain the necessity for turning Norman from one side to the other and I had to explain to them that he could not tolerate being placed on either side and had not been able to tolerate this since falling ill in January 2013. As, with other professionals in the past, both found this difficult to understand or accept and went on to explain the importance of positioning, especially, shoulders, hips, knees, ankles. Although this clarified that the positioning we had been putting Norman into since the morning he had woken me by shouting "help", was correct, it was extremely interesting to hear it voiced by specialists. Their knowledge was also extremely useful with regard to what cushions and pillows we could use and where in the bed in order to ensure that we did not compromise the benefits of the air mattress. The OTs then went on to say, yet again, that Norman needed to be turned and despite voicing my disapproval strongly, insisted on trying. Yet again to my dismay, it was only Norman that suffered from people refusing to listen to me (clearly when it comes to the NHS I have no voice). Up until this point I had managed to keep the OTs gentle and aware of not moving Norman too quickly or extravagantly but now they were on a mission. They both took hold of him and started to almost "toss" him to the left and then to the right using a double-length bolster pillow. Norman's face became contorted; he started to scream and was clearly distressed but both OTs were deaf to this. I had to voice his distress and pain on his behalf and *shouted* to ensure I was heard "Stop – look what you are doing; look at his face, listen to him scream, you cannot put Norman through this." The OTs stopped and finally accepted that they were not going to place Norman on either side. Despite this, it was a very useful visit as it confirmed that what we had been doing was the correct positioning. It was just a shame, yet again, that the visit took place approximately ten months after discharge instead of one month after discharge – and I had to ask myself; "Do they not use this knowledge in the nursing home?" Sadly, however, this did seem to be the way of things. So much knowledge is out there but it is extremely difficult to access it in a timely manner, before it is too late.

Within a short while from our visit to the neurologist, we received a telephone call from our local hospice, and an appointment was made for a palliative doctor to come out to visit us. She came in and spoke to Norman. Norman recognised her genuine interest in World War I and II planes and although did not engage in a conversation with her, his facial expressions were more attentive than usual. The palliative doctor visited a couple of times and complimented us on the way we were caring for Norman. She referred to the job I had taken on for Norman as being the Project Manager and reckoned it would be a great asset if we were able to duplicate what I was doing for him and put more "me's" out into the community to look after other people. I have to say, it may sound selfish but I readily accepted that compliment. The experiences over the previous months were beginning to leave me mentally battered and bruised. So many times, I had said to Kevin "I understand people not wanting to or unable to help me, but if only they would stop putting so many obstructions in my way." During one visit she asked if I knew about the facility to have a "matron" working for us. I replied "No" and she explained that if a matron was allocated to Norman it would save a lot of stress as the matron would organise meetings/nursing etc. on my behalf and may reduce the need for mental capacity tests. She offered to look into this for me and said she would come back to me and naturally, I thanked her. Yet another facility available but not readily offered.

On Monday morning, the 2nd March 2015 I came downstairs and went straight into Norman as I always did about 7 to 7.30 a.m. To my horror Norman's face was yet again contorted and near to tears. Clearly he was very stressed and scared. I could see him trying to speak but no noise was coming out. I reassured him as best I could and told him it did not matter if he could not speak, just to raise his right hand the best he can and we will know what he wants. I called Peter and went to ring the doctor. The doctor came and felt that Norman had suffered a small stroke sometime during the night but the doctor did not feel that there was anything to be gained by taking Norman to hospital. With the benefit of hindsight, I believe that this was the day that Norman entered into "End of Life". From this day forward it was more and more difficult to coax Norman to eat or drink and within a couple of weeks we were extremely worried. Visits to Speech and Therapy were increased but to no avail. By the third week in March I decided that we would have to order soft and pureed food from Wiltshire Foods as this was the only way to obtain the correct texture for Norman and also to ensure a varied diet. These meals were excellent and helped both Peter and Cassandra to ensure that Norman ate properly.

He did not appear to be responding though, we were all becoming increasingly concerned about the amount of food and drink he was taking on board and how sleepy and unresponsive he was so I contacted the doctor and told him. Urine tract infections often cause people to be very sleepy but the doctor did not think that was Norman's problem, but as a precaution advised us to take a urine sample for analysis which we did. A couple of days later, the doctor contacted me to say that Norman did have a UTI but it was one which would not respond to normal antibiotics. I asked the way forward and the doctor explained that the drugs needed were hospital drugs and only normally administered in hospital by intravenous injection. Both the doctor and I were very worried about admitting Norman to hospital as our fears were we would never be able to discharge him home again. The doctor explained that it may be possible for the local NHS Provide Nursing team to administer the hospital drugs by intravenous injection at home and he would look into it and come back to me.

It took the doctor ten days to organise the medication that Norman required and, yet again, the only one who suffered was Norman, but nevertheless the doctor rang back to say that he was just waiting delivery of the drug and the five-day treatment would commence on Thursday – it was now Tuesday.

The next day, I was driving to work when my mobile rang. I parked the car and answered the mobile. It was the local NHS Community Nurse Manager. She said that she understood that Norman needed a five-day intravenous drug and I confirmed this. She then went on to explain that before this procedure could possibly take place she and the doctor would have to come out and carry out a "mental capacity" test. I was livid. Steam was coming out of my ears. I told her that this had been arranged by our doctor to which she replied that he was now on holiday for a couple of days and another doctor would attend with her. I asked why, when a doctor had arranged the procedure and had seen Norman, but she insisted on Norman being subjected to a "mental capacity" test prior to the medication being administered. I asked "Why is a nurse able to over-rule a doctor?" She replied "It is necessary". So yet again realising that I had no voice I asked her to confirm that the only way forward was for the nurse and doctor to come out and (in my opinion "cruelly") subject Norman, who was particularly unwell to *yet another* "mental capacity" test. She said "Yes." I replied: "Ok, so when Norman fails the "mental capacity" test which he will, what will happen?" She replied: "He will still be given the five-day intravenous drug under 'best interests'". (Another example of no compassion, empathy, or understanding, of Norman's wellbeing and psychological state – let's just torture him, shall we?!) I asked "What time?" and she replied "2.00 p.m. this afternoon."

So 2 p.m. that afternoon came and they both arrived for the mental capacity test. The doctor was extremely quick. Norman failed the mental capacity test but they agreed the need for the drug under "best interests". The nurse, however, made herself comfortable in our lounge for two hours and we found ourselves being interrogated. At one point Kevin became very cross which was extremely unusual as he is very laid back and I was the one telling him to calm down. When she finally left he remarked "What was that all about?" and I replied "Our motives and intentions regarding caring for Norman have just been tested and scrutinised to the nth degree." For me, it is cruel and a form of torture to continually subject a seriously ill individual, who has already many many times said that he wants his sister to look after him, to mental capacity test after mental capacity test, but unfortunately the only way to avoid this is to obtain Lasting Power of Attorney for Health and Welfare and I still wonder if even this would have helped – but, I do know, it is wrong and I also know that anyone else with any sense of compassion seeing their family member constantly subjected to these tests and the terrible affects it has on their mental state would also know – *it is wrong!*

The next day the intravenous medication started and for Norman I am sure that the insertion of the canola was very painful – certainly observing his face and having no voice at all now he clearly was very scared. I stayed with him throughout the administration of the drug and held his hand. Overall the five days went well with no complications. However, it had little effect and Norman did not improve.

Within a week, Norman was suddenly violently sick without warning. It was now out of hours and we were very worried regarding the lack of fluids he was taking on and his general wellbeing. I was very concerned. What if Norman was suffering from a bug or flu and I did not get him the hospital treatment he needed and he died when he did not need to? But if he went into hospital, I would be unlikely to discharge him. I agonised and finally made the decision to call an ambulance and he was admitted immediately.

Accompanying him to hospital, I kept telling everyone and anyone who was listening (or not listening as the case may be!) that Norman was here to be rehydrated as a full care package was in place at home. Of course, I was wasting my breath but I had to do something. Whilst waiting in the corridor for Norman to be seen, a young nurse came over with hospital arm tags and placed one on Norman and said "Right, now you belong to us." It was such an innocent remark on her part just making polite conversation but, to me, it rang so true. It made me think and realise that throughout this journey with Norman it had been a continuous fight for me, only his sister, to care for him. It seemed that once you fell ill you lost your status as a human being and became "property" of the NHS which again highlighted the importance of Lasting Power of Attorney for Health and Welfare for those who want a family member to have a say in their care and/or medical treatment.

The next morning, Peter went to the hospital and found Norman in a distressed state. Although he was better being hydrated the hospital had not positioned him correctly and he was slumped to his left with his head buried in his body. Peter took charge and positioned him correctly making Norman much more comfy. I had been on the telephone to our doctor asking for him to write to the hospital confirming that a full care package was in place and once hydrated Norman should be discharged home. The doctor agreed readily to do this for me and said the letter would be waiting on reception for me to collect. I also contacted the palliative doctor and asked her to do the same. Fortunately she was visiting the hospital that day and said she would meet me there. I also contacted the secretary of the Medical Director of the hospital and reminded her of who we were, i.e. the hospital had given Norman septicaemia June 13 and asked that the Medical Director arrange for his discharge once hydrated.

Thankfully as I rushed out of the house to make my way to the hospital, I remembered to pick up the folder containing all of the paperwork of the care package that we had compiled. On arrival at the hospital I went to see Norman. The tissue viability nurse was present, examining Norman together with Peter. The tissue viability nurse was giving Peter a hard time regarding the state of Norman's skin. The hospital had not placed Norman on an air mattress, nor had they taken care of his positioning so overnight his skin breakdown had significantly worsened. Peter was trying to explain but the nurse would not listen. As soon as I entered, the nurse started on me and initially I started to react and found myself in an argument as the skin viability nurse was far from happy. The palliative doctor arrived together with the head nurse that the Medical Director had sent and both stood listening to the game of tennis that the skin viability nurse and I were having regarding the treatment of Norman's skin. Looking across to Norman I could see him lifting his right hand slightly, which I knew to mean "I want to go home." Eventually, it came to me and I asked the skin viability nurse to wait and listen. I explained that at home Norman was on an air mattress. He said he could get one. "Yes," I said, "But you cannot get a purpose-made tall shower chair, a ceiling hoist, a Comfy Chair and a wheelchair." I explained our care package included moving Norman regularly using all of this equipment and his skin had worsened significantly since being admitted.

The nurse went quiet and said defiantly "OK but I will be submitting my report and here is a copy." I took it and thanked him. Clearly, he was still not happy at the state of Norman's skin. It was now the turn of the head nurse (who the Medical Director had sent) to attack me as he was horrified at the idea of Norman being discharged and had already made arrangements for him to be transferred to another ward. Another heated discussion took place. The head nurse stated: "Norman needs to see Speech and Therapy." Referring to my care package folder I answered "Yes, Norman saw so and so on such and such date." The nurse then said "Norman needs to see a dietician," and I replied, "Yes booked for such and such date." This went on for a few more questions and, finally, the palliative doctor spoke up and reported that she had been to our house and described the care package in place for Norman as being excellent. Not wishing to give in without a fight, the head nurse then said "Ok, Norman can be discharged provided he drinks a glass of water." Now I was more than a little anxious. Would Norman be able to drink a glass of water? All throughout our discussions I had looked over towards Norman and his right hand had kept raising an inch saying "I want to go home." I looked straight at Norman and said, "I am really sorry Norman but you must drink this glass of water in order for us to take you home." Despite how ill he was he started to drink. To this day, it upsets me to remember the determination and distress on his face but he knew what he had to do and he swallowed every drop despite the difficulty he was experiencing. The nurse said "Ok. I'll arrange transport," to which I replied "Don't worry, our mobility vehicle is downstairs." We gave the head nurse no opportunity to think of another challenge and immediately hoisted Norman into his wheelchair, Peter probably broke all speed restrictions in the hospital as he pushed him through the corridors and into the mobility car. Finally, we had escaped and Peter drove us all home.

The re-hydration had made a slight difference to Norman and Duxford was only two weeks away and Peter was looking forward to taking him there. However, daily, Norman started to deteriorate. I spoke to the doctor and asked if he could receive hydration at home. I said that we wanted to take him to Duxford as it was Norman's passion. The doctor confirmed that it was not possible to hydrate him at home but the amount he had had should last ten days. Within a day or so we could not persuade Norman to eat or drink anything. I rang the palliative doctor and our doctor. Arrangements would be made to deliver highly-nutritional drinks for Norman. Every day we were waiting and every day we seemed to see him disappear further from us. Peter and Cassandra doubled up to care for him. Within a week, his breathing became particularly shallow. Tearfully, I rang the palliative doctor Tuesday evening out of hours and asked for help. The person who answered the telephone was very kind, suggested we changed Norman's position and said she would ask the palliative doctor to call. I spoke to the palliative doctor and our doctor the next day and explained through tears that we seemed to be losing Norman. Neither doctor seemed to comprehend the seriousness of the situation. The palliative doctor said she would visit in a week's time. I was extremely anxious. I explained that I did not know whether or not he was in any pain. Both doctors agreed to order painkillers ready for collection but I believe that neither doctor appreciated that Norman was dying. The painkillers were never collected. That night I took Norman a cup of tea in at 10 p.m. He was now laying to his right looking out of the window which he had done for the past three days. Up until then, he had laid towards the left facing towards the door. I put the cup to his lips and he took two small sips and closed his eyes. I put the lights out and left his room. That night I could hear Norman snoring. It was about 6 a.m. and I went downstairs and stood outside his door. Should I go in? I stayed outside and at 7 a.m. he stopped snoring and so I went upstairs. I came back down at 7.30 a.m. and went into his room to say good morning. Immediately, I could see that his chest was not rising. Norman had died. I had lost my older brother aged 66 - 2 years

5 months after finding him collapsed. To me this was young. Up until his collapse I had never considered him dying before the age of 70/80 plus – after all we all live longer now, don't we? But, here I was, he had gone, I no longer had a brother.

I rang 999 and through tears told them that my brother had died. Sympathetically they asked me the questions they needed the answers to. "Did he have a no resuscitation order?" I answered "Yes, he did this had been arranged on discharge from hospital ten days ago". They asked "Are you sure?" and I went to the documentation and read it to them. I was told that someone would be with me shortly. She arrived and told me that she was qualified to recognise death but could not pronounce death and I would have to call the doctor.

I telephoned the doctor. By now it was approximately 9 a.m. I explained to the receptionist what had happened and she asked me to hold. When she came back she said that all of the doctors were busy taking morning surgery and a doctor would be with me at approximately 2 p.m. I thanked her and put the telephone down. It is difficult to describe my feelings, I felt panicked, cold, numb, tearful, shocked and, initially, wanted Norman collected as soon as possible. Just leaving him there, dead, seemed somehow disrespectful to him but then I started to reflect on my brief experiences whilst working for a funeral director and started to think through the situation from a totally different aspect. It was Norman's house; so he was no longer with us in body but that was no reason to kick him out of his own house. Suddenly, the situation took on a totally different perspective and I felt comforted that he was still here and I could "pop-in" and see him at my leisure. Whilst working for the funeral directors, people would call to see their family member in the chapel to say their final goodbyes and invariably it was a short encounter. Now I had hours to reflect and say goodbye. I look back on that time now and actually find quite a lot of comfort in it and it still brings tears to my eyes. It was right for Norman not to be rushed out of the house the minute he died. He would never have purposefully hurt me when he was alive so he was not going to hurt me once he had died, him staying with us for a couple of hours after death was respectful and an expression of our love for him.

The doctor came and certified Norman as dead and shortly afterwards he was collected by the funeral directors. Again it is so difficult to express the feelings as he was taken out of the house for the last time. Once the door was closed, Kevin and I were left in this now empty house. Since moving in it had been a busy environment with people coming and going at all times of day and our private life non-existent. What do we do now? That interim period of readjustment is horrendous. I did not want to stay in the house. I did not want to go out. I sat staring into space; I did not want to do this. I did not want to occupy myself carrying out any jobs. Finally, we decided to take Jet out for a walk and reflect upon the last few days and the days ahead.

When I reflect, I find it difficult to understand why neither of the two doctors nor the hospital, realised that Norman was so near to death. To some degree it irritates me that people who die from a well-known and understood illness receive palliative care and their last days/hours are well catered for, but I truly believe that for Norman only having those he knew present was the best and kindest way for him to pass away.

I do still have two pleasant memories of May 2015 just before Norman passed away as Kevin, Cassandra and I together with Jet managed to take him to a local country house and I sat with him in the Great Hall whilst Kevin and Cassandra looked around the rooms upstairs. We took it in turn to push him around the grounds and whilst I was pushing I suddenly stopped and said, "OK, I need a smile before I can continue" and went round to look at Norman's face and was greeted with a cheeky grin. Probably ten to fourteen days before he passed away the three of us took him to a local annual World War II day. His head was down most of the time and his eyes were closed but driving home, suddenly he looked up and I remarked "Oh, you've joined us then."

Chapter 7
Norman's Funeral

In response to my telephone call, the funeral directors contacted me to make the necessary arrangements and, as we were not a religious family, I decided to go for a humanist funeral with a touch of religion. Arrangements were made for the humanist to call. She was a lovely considerate person and started to ask background questions in order to form an opinion as to a suitable service for Norman. When my dad had died I had not been involved with any of the arrangements and when my mum died ten years ago, Norman and I made the arrangements. Very quickly, however, it became evident that funerals had changed considerably over the past ten years and it was more acceptable to celebrate the person's life. The humanist wanted sufficient information to write a Eulogy and gently probed me for answers. A cold shiver came over me as I did not want to answer all these questions. Simply, to bring the meeting to an end I told her that I would write the Eulogy myself. Surprised at this, she asked sympathetically "Are you sure?" and shortly afterwards reiterated this question "Are you sure?", and I replied "Yes." The truth was, I was thinking no further than I wanted this meeting to end which was no disrespect to her, she was lovely, I was just not coping. I was feeling very emotional and tearful. I think it hurts so much more when it is a sister or brother who dies. They are a similar age group. We are conditioned to accept the death of our parents, providing of course it is a natural death. But I, for one, had never considered my brother not only dying so young but dying from such a dreadful disease causing such considerable suffering and it is almost slightly selfish in that by dying he has affected my life as I no longer have close family members. Of course, I have Kevin my husband who is very important but I no longer have close blood family members. It is a sharp reminder of my own immortality. Nothing lasts forever. Our life is only a small and trivial chapter in a very large book.

Yet again calling upon my experiences working for a funeral director, I realised that my emotions were perfectly normal and part of the grieving process. Everyone is subjected to the grieving process but rarely in the same order or to the same timescale. However, I did not have time to wallow in my own grief; I needed to write a Eulogy and had no idea where to begin. I started to regret by snap decision but equally could not bring myself to ask the humanist back and sat in front of my computer with a blank page. One of her questions had burned its way into my memory – "What will you miss most about your brother?" I started to think of this over and over again. The answer was, I knew no matter what I needed, where I was, how long I needed him – whatever I asked of Norman the answer was an unconditional "Yes." Norman was my brother and we lived our own, different and separate, lives but if I needed him for whatever reason, he would be there without fail and as quickly as possible for as long as I needed him. He was 100% reliable and I knew it. This formed the basis of my Eulogy and it grew from there. The Eulogy, I think, was the most difficult thing I have encountered in my life. I could not stop the tears cascading down my face to the extent that I could not see what I was typing and typed blindly – thank goodness for my training as a "touch typist"! I could not control the tears but it proved to be the most rewarding thing I have ever done. I think it also helped enormously with the grieving process, it was one of the last things I could do for Norman.

The next difficulty was finding the music for the funeral. I decided to take a risk. After all we did not expect many people to come so it felt like "my funeral for my brother". We never expressed our feelings when he was alive, at least this gave me the opportunity now albeit arguably rather late. Norman had been extremely passionate about his World War planes especially the Sally B. Could I obtain a soundtrack of the Sally B or something similar flying? I started to formulate the idea of Norman entering the chapel to the familiar sound of something he loved like Sally B. It would be like he was attending his last air show, not his funeral. I was not completely confident though that those attending would understand and asked the humanist to comment on the sounds once Norman had entered.

The next music sound was easy, Norman and I had chosen "Amazing Grace" played by the Dragoon Guards for my mother's funeral and being respectful to both my mother and Norman I chose this music to mark our final goodbye to Norman.

The humanist had suggested having a minute's silence in the middle of the service for those attending to reflect and remember Norman. He also loved all wildlife and fishing. I asked one of his fishing companions if he had any photos of Norman fishing. Ant had been friends with Norman since their secondary school days and he promised to email me a couple. I decided to print on the back of the order of service a photograph of Norman holding his catch of the day. When it came to the time of the minute's silence, I asked that the humanist refer those attending to turn to the back page and think of Norman fishing. We did not have silence; we played sounds of common song birds. The reflection was thinking of Norman fishing whilst listening to song birds singing.

The day of the funeral arrived and I was only expecting a few people. Norman had never married and so did not have any family of his own. As I looked around I saw people gathering. Norman was right – his friends from his many hobbies, fishing, photography, and Bomber Group, did attend his funeral. His previous next-door neighbours were also there, together with his business colleagues. Several of my friends also came who knew me more than Norman but were there to respect him and to support me at this sad time. I remain eternally grateful and thankful to my friends who attended in support of me. People can be so kind and thoughtful. One of my regrets is that clearly I had not had sufficient service of order sheets printed but we coped by sharing them. After the service, so many people came to me and commented on what a perfect and thoughtful send-off it was for Norman. In fact they surprised me by coming back to the house again for reflection and refreshments. It highlights that the funeral of a person is really for those that are left to take comfort in remembering the passing of their friend or family in the best way possible. Norman's friends and colleagues stayed sometime looking through the photo albums that I had put out in remembrance of him. A funeral does not have to be something you endure it can, in its way, help you through the grieving process and honour and celebrate the life of the person who has passed away.

Referring back, again, to the time I spent working for funeral directors, I had been surprised at how many people left their family member's ashes with the funeral director. Not only for a short or long time but, sometimes, forever as they were never collected. For some reason, this practice appalled me. It was so disrespectful. The task of honouring and celebrating an individual's life is not complete until the ashes have been taken care of. There was no way, I was going to leave Norman's ashes at the funeral directors and I arranged their collection immediately. Now, however, my "righteous" self has been challenged. My dad's ashes had been interred by Mum arranging it and Norman and I had arranged interment of Mum's and it isn't possible to place Norman with either Mum or Dad. So my dilemma, what do I do? I could scatter them at his favourite fishing place and discussed this with Ant and Terence. I could take them and place them at an appropriate place at the Bomber Museum where Norman spent so much time. I could bury them just outside his bedroom at home and he would remain with us (unless we moved). It saddens me to admit, that I am no longer so "righteous" as even three years after his death,

I cannot bring myself to place them somewhere permanently and they remain stored in our garage – an outstanding part of these reflections which, one day, I will have to accept and deal with. A psychologist would probably say that I have not yet accepted Norman's death but I think it is a female trait – I just keep changing my mind!

A month or two after the funeral I was contacted by the Chairman of the Bomber Group. He told me that the Group wanted to put two memorials up to remember two people who had contributed so greatly to them and one of these people was Norman. The Chairman commented on how respected and liked Norman had been and they were missing the relentless hard work and energy he had spent ensuring the continuance of the Group. The memorial would be a bench and plaque to be unveiled at the next American Reunion Day and would I come along and unveil it. Again, lots of emotion, honoured, choked, and thrilled, that Norman was so highly thought of – also sad that this had been a large part of his life that I had been only on the very fringe of. The answer was "Yes, when?"

Kevin, I, Jet and a friend, travelled to Suffolk on the day of the American Reunion. Once there we had to feast our eyes on the number of people attending and enjoying themselves and the amount of work the committee had put in to ensure this was a successful day. The time came for the unveiling and luckily for me, the other person's bench was unveiled first which gave me time to think about what I was going to say. My mind was blank. I tried harder to think. My mind was blank. I had not a clue what to say. In fact, my vocabulary consisted of two words, "Thank you."

It was time for me to unveil Norman's bench and I went to stand in front of a huge number of people, their eyes all upon me. Suddenly, a brainwave. I decided to talk from the heart. I explained that although this was not my hobby, I was so touched and moved that Norman had been such an important part of their unique family unit. I thanked all present for the best wishes Norman and I had received since the day he had collapsed until the day he had died and sympathy cards at his funeral. I looked at my friend and tears were falling down her face. I had to look away as I was still holding it together. After the unveiling, several people came up to me and complimented me on my speech. They then went on to say what a lovely person Norman had been and how much he had helped the committee. He had become their photographer and had taken several beautiful photographs. He had also started their website and printed calendars, together with supplying key rings and other mementoes to sell and most importantly had spoken to a friend who ran a small brewery and arranged for the Red Feather Club, which was the officers' club, to have its own beer. We all went in for a fantastic cream tea and cakes. Jet's mouth was watering!

After our tea, a few people came up to express their sympathy and I also learnt of a couple of chilling stories which I had no idea of. Apparently Norman was always first to arrive at the committee meetings despite travelling the furthest, approximately a two- hour drive. He had been on the committee for some time and knew this journey like the back of his hand. This particular time, he did not arrive until halfway through the meeting and was clearly distressed. The Chairman tried to talk to Norman, saying that they had been very worried about him but all the Chairman could glean from him is that he had got lost and had become disorientated. Another person told me that Norman had called into them unexpectedly – again because he was lost and did not know his way home. Norman, once had told me that he was sick on the way home and I had asked "Did you eat something that disagreed with you?" but he did not answer. With the benefit of hindsight, I can only surmise that these were early episodes of the onset of his brain disease – mini-strokes affecting him for a short space of time. Someone else had told me that they had thought Norman had been drinking when he answered the front door to them as his speech was slurred. Unfortunately, neither Kevin nor I had witnessed any of these symptoms/episodes. If only someone had told me!

Elizabeth Orr

Chapter 8
It should have been better!

It was the right decision to discharge Norman. His quality of life was far better at home than in the neurological nursing home and despite all of the stresses experienced, neither Kevin nor I regret our decision in any way. I'm sure that had Norman been left in the neurological nursing home he would have slipped into his own world reciting "Boo."

My regrets are the length of time it took us to discharge Norman – the time left to him was precious as his health declined daily – but no one but us recognised this or even cared, the attitude we witnessed was "tomorrow will do". It also took us far too long to get his care package right. Based on our experiences, it would appear that the care sector is not equipped to deal with individuals as ill as Norman at home. The only way to cope is to employ carers direct and compile your own personal care package tailored to the individual.

My learning curve was vertical and I did the best I could but it could have, and should have, been better. It is incredible how much information and knowledge is out there but (in my opinion) the organisations in the respective sectors (medical, care, financial and legal) all need to be more transparent, and readily accessible. They most certainly need to be more helpful and less obstructive. Perhaps it is down to not having the correct paperwork in place (e.g. Lasting Powers of Attorney for both Property & Finance and Health & Welfare), or perhaps

141

the organisations should buy hearing aids so that they hear our voices! Most certainly they should look up the meaning of their own sayings "best interests" and "duty of care" and adhere to them.

Whenever I hear an aeroplane now, I look up and think of Norman. We still have Jet, the black Labrador we bought for Norman, and he is an adorable dog in every way. Occasionally, however, when Jet is being a nuisance wanting his "tenth" walk of the day or his "tenth" meal of the day, I hear Norman's voice saying "It's good for you!", a favourite saying of his.

Norman, plenty of people were more than willing to care for you but not many could cope with your complex and complicated care needs. Few possessed the necessary empathy and understanding of the serious conditions you were suffering from such as brain disease, general neuropathy and rheumatoid arthritis. The high majority, simply, did not have the required skills probably due to lack of training or even possibly due to the industry's low pay. Our journey together should have been much easier and less tortuous for us both but I can say with hand on heart Norman, we cared passionately about your quality of life during your final journey and are so pleased that we tried and although it took far too long to get it right - finally:-

WE LEARNT HOW TO CARE FOR YOU

PART TWO

What Should Have Been Better?

If Only I Had Known

It is fair to say that this experience has changed my outlook on life and beliefs considerably especially towards the importance of Lasting Power of Attorney documentation and the NHS. What perhaps has not changed is my "principled" self – right is right and wrong is wrong and, for me, so much of what happened on our journey was wrong. As an individual, there are many aspects well outside my influence or control and to which I can not make a difference (nursing ratios, medical care, skill and training of carers, more timely access to specialists and knowledge of vital services/facilities available). Maybe, just maybe, someone who can make a difference will read this book and take action – here's hoping.

There were, however, points well within my control (or Norman's control) which would have made a huge difference – the most important being Lasting Powers of Attorney for Property & Finance and Health & Welfare. What I can do, is share my experiences with you regarding the following very important and, for me, hugely stressful, areas encountered on my journey caring for Norman. Perhaps this, in turn, may influence your decision to raise these documents for yourself or encourage a family member to do so in a timely manner. For me, Lasting Power of Attorney papers are like an insurance policy, you only think about them when the worst happens but based on my experience, not having to deal with the "fall out" far outweighs the inconvenience and modest cost of raising and registering them.

1. Lasting Power of Attorney (LPA) for Property & Financial Affairs

Throughout life, I think it is human nature not to take notice or think of things unless they cross your path or touch you personally. Kevin and I had made a Will several years ago and, thankfully, so had Norman, but none of us had considered or discussed Lasting Power of Attorney for either Property & Finance or Health & Welfare but the importance of these documents plagued me throughout Norman's illness.

Initially, Norman's finances were easy for me to cope with. The house bills were paid by direct debit and he was still able to make a signature and so would sign a few cheques for me for insurances, etc. Even after six months and there was talk about Norman going to a neurological nursing home I still did not want to step on his toes regarding his finances. I kept thinking he would get better. Norman and I spoke about his current account and he agreed that I should be added as a signatory. This was very easy, I obtained the forms, completed, signed and submitted, them to the high street bank and once processed I was able to sign on Norman's account which was fortuitous as it was not long after this that he lost the ability to sign.

The difficulty came when we decided to sell our house and Norman's bungalow in order to buy a suitable house to enable us to discharge Norman from the nursing home. I contacted his Financial Advisor who managed Norman's money in an "investment bank". During our conversations the Financial Advisor insisted that we use the investment bank's solicitors despite my having already completed the documents. Not wishing to be awkward (and probably naively) I agreed. A meeting was arranged with the solicitors and after the solicitor held a one-to-one meeting with Norman, he announced to me that Norman had not only requested that I be one of the Attorneys for the Property & Financial Affairs LPA but also his Financial Advisor (are bells ringing yet?). At the time, I was desperate to get the finances set up in order to buy the house -

my thoughts were only with Norman. The last thing I wanted to do was quiz Norman or be awkward and so I agreed. I was also aware that if I had an accident or fell ill, then there was someone else who could act on his behalf.

The documentation appointing both the Financial Advisor and myself as Attorneys was raised and submitted. The investment bank solicitor's cost for this was much higher than other solicitors but although aware of this point, again I accepted it. The solicitor called a meeting to distribute the Lasting Power of Attorney for Property & Financial Affairs documents to us both and also outlined additional fees which I refused to pay.

Within the next few days, I submitted the Lasting Power of Attorney documents for Property & Financial Affairs to those organisations that I needed to and I assumed (wrongly) that by giving the Financial Advisor an original copy at the solicitor's meeting, the investment bank had also been notified.

During the next six months from January 2014 to June 2014, my dealings with the Financial Advisor were, from my point of view, stressful to say the least. Despite the conflict of interest, he remained Norman's Financial Advisor and controlled Norman's finances. By June 2014, I could not understand why – not only did the Financial Advisor ignore my requests for transfer of funds, but he also chose to reduce the amount of a transfer requested by letter which I had asked Norman to sign. Finally, after ringing the investment bank's office, I found out that the Financial Advisor had not registered the Lasting Power of Attorney for Property & Financial Affairs. After raising a rumpus, I was asked to submit the documents myself to the investment bank and as a result of this, another Financial Advisor was appointed to Norman's account. Dealings still remained fraught though, because whenever I dealt with the investment bank, their staff would inform me that they would have to run it past Norman's initial Financial Advisor first as he was Joint Attorney. There were other issues as well which I have chosen not to go into detail here but, effectively, despite being Norman's Financial Attorney for Financial Affairs I had no say with the investment bankers. Norman's finances were controlled by the original Financial Advisor who had been appointed Attorney by the investment bank's solicitors.

In January 2015 (five months before Norman's death) it was even more difficult for Norman to pronounce words but as my dealings with his original Financial Advisor/Attorney were as stressful as ever I decided to ask him. I said "Norman, how did it come about for 'Walter' to become your other Attorney? Did you ask for him, or did the solicitor suggest?" You would have had to be there to appreciate the effort Norman put into answering. He struggled but finally said "Soli..ci..tor su..gge..s..ted." I am so pleased that I asked because his answer not only informed me that he had not requested/wanted "Walter" to be an Attorney, the solicitor had; but also that Norman wanted me to know this fact.

I remember one time in particular whilst walking around the grounds of the neurological nursing home greeting another visitor. We had smiled several times at each other but this time we stopped and spoke. He told me that his wife was there after suffering a serious stroke and that they lived in London. He was now travelling down regularly to visit his wife and was finding the length and cost of the journey difficult. He then went on to explain that he was in the process of trying to move somewhere nearer the neurological nursing home so that he could be with his wife but he had encountered difficulties in selling their existing house as he did not have Lasting Power of Attorney for Property & Financial Affairs and the property was registered in both their names and he was unable to obtain her authority/agreement to sell.

2. Lasting Power of Attorney for Health & Welfare

This document is perhaps the least discussed but in a way the most important. I had asked the solicitor appointed by the investment bank during our first meeting about Lasting Power of Attorney for Health & Welfare and he replied that we should consider it in the future. To this day, I do not understand why the solicitor did not complete both Lasting Powers of Attorney at the same time. I have since learnt that it is normal practice within the legal sector to do so.

Sadly, the only person who suffered by not having Lasting Power of Attorney for Health & Welfare was, yet again, Norman. He was constantly subjected to mental capacity test after mental capacity test because each test is only valid for each subject tested. From Norman's point of view he had said several times that he wanted me to represent him, so why did he keep being asked the same questions? Even when you are well, you do not like people interrogating you. The medical sector do not appear to care regarding the psychological effects it has on patients when they are subjected to these tests, especially when the patient is told that they have failed (as Norman was) when, in fact, he had supplied the correct answer.

Once Norman was home and I became more aware of the importance of Lasting Power of Attorney for Health & Welfare and the effects it was having on him, I did try to obtain it but, again sadly, despite the solicitor believing that Norman was fully aware of what we were referring to and its repercussions, she would not raise the documents unless she received a letter from his doctor confirming he had mental capacity and the doctor refused to furnish her with such a letter. My voice therefore continued to fall on deaf ears making the caring for Norman significantly more difficult and Norman continued to suffer needlessly. It is cruel and a form of torture especially as so often he would pass or fail depending upon the answer those that were testing him wanted. If it was beneficial to them for him to pass he would pass, if it was beneficial for him to fail, he would fail.

3. Probate – Obstructive "investment bank"

Thankfully, Norman had made a Will and had left it in a place which could easily be found and I had a copy of it. The

Will named me as joint executor with the named solicitors. I contacted the solicitors upon Norman's death and made an appointment to visit them. I can only assume that I was particularly sensitive during our meeting as yet again my impression was one of "greed" looking to obtain as much money as possible from the account. During our conversations, the solicitors said that probate would be relatively easy as there appeared to be only about four letters to write but the cost would be a percentage of Norman's estate which was several thousand pounds. The solicitor also started to ramble on as to whether or not oil left in the oil tank for the central heating system for the house was subject to inheritance tax. I left the meeting exhausted, frustrated, and angered, yet again – it must be me! However, on the way home Kevin (unusually) spoke and commented adversely about the meeting – perhaps it wasn't me!

Coincidentally, I spoke to Terence who had a good idea of the funds involved and he told me that he had completed probate for his mother and saw no reason why I should not do this myself; which started me thinking and, although I had no idea of what I was letting myself in for, I decided to contact the solicitors and ask them to put a hold on any work regarding Norman's estate. A partner of the firm responded surprisingly quickly by contacting me the next day. After a long expensive conversation she agreed to forward to me options together with their respective costs for obtaining probate. My mind started to work overtime. Norman's estate was very straightforward – the solicitors had said so themselves – only four letters. I held qualifications in accounts, secretarial and computers, and most of the information I would have to supply to the solicitors myself anyway, they would then instruct a junior to carry out the legwork and a senior would only spend an hour or two reviewing the file. I decided to be the junior myself and contacted the partner of the solicitor's firm asking that if I completed the file, would they review it for me and to my surprise they agreed. As they were not going to carry out the work in house, they expressed their wish to withdraw from being executors and I could understand this but asked that their status be changed to "Power Reserved" rather than deleted as, if I fell ill or had an accident, they would be able to step in to complete Norman's estate and the solicitors agreed.

I ordered the respective forms from the HMRC and spoke to them when needed. HMRC were particularly helpful. When contacting the investment bank asking for the relevant figures, true to form they were obstructive making it extremely obvious that they were not happy dealing with me, they wanted to deal direct with the solicitors and had trouble in accepting that I was the only Executor – the status of the solicitors was now "Power Reserved". The investment bank made life very difficult for me and continued to be as obstructive and awkward as possible. The high street bank involved could not have been more understanding, compassionate or helpful. I compiled a probate file completing all the paperwork and asked the solicitors to review this on my behalf which they did and their fees for this were only a small percentage of the original figure quoted.

The only difficulty was that inheritance tax had to be paid to HMRC before probate would be granted. The high street bank could not be more helpful and paid the amount I asked direct to HMRC but this was not sufficient and so I contacted the investment bank who could not have been more obstructive if they tried. Despite several telephone calls, exchange of letters, emails, etc., the investment bank refused to transfer any money even though the transaction was zero risk as it was a transfer from a cash account, and not investments which would have to be sold. Luckily, I had sufficient savings of my own and so was able to fulfil HMRC's requirements of paying all of the inheritance tax before probate.

The investment bank was obviously shocked when I delivered the probate papers to them and, in addition to this, I had managed to complete probate within six months despite the house we bought in Norman's name being part of the inheritance. Apparently, it is very unusual to complete probate on time within six months especially when a house is involved as its valuation has to be agreed by HMRC.

Complaint Re Investment Bank

After probate had been granted and the monies received into my bank account from the investment bank, I decided to write a complaint letter to their CEO to give him the opportunity of sharing my journey with them since Norman had collapsed. Their reply included that they had not registered the Lasting Power of Attorney for Property & Financial Affairs presented to them in January 2014 until I forced them to in June 2014 because it *had not been necessary*. Eventually, my complaint went to the Ombudsman and their arbitrator found the investment bank to be in the wrong and asked for an unconditional letter of apology to be forwarded to me. In addition, the arbitrator informed me that some of the points raised in my complaint regarding procedures, had been taken on board by the investment bank and procedures would be reviewed – who knows – but we do know that if people do not complain, nothing will change.

I do know that the financial planners I use personally reacted to my experience by updating their existing Vulnerable Clients' Policy to include specific references to managing best outcomes for the "critically ill" including a strong focus on arranging Lasting Powers of Attorney documents for both Property & Finance and Health & Welfare.

I have agonised over whether or not to include this chapter in the book because, perhaps, our experience and Norman's dreadful brain disease is rare, but my mind keeps coming back to the fact that although medical science has improved tremendously resulting in hospitals saving more lives, it is not until that life has been saved that they know how much of that person is left – that is to say how brain-damaged are they?

Also, my experience has been that investment banks are far less accommodating (bordering obstructive) and helpful than high street banks when the worst happens – ***why?***

With the Benefit of Hindsight

For sure, with the benefit of hindsight, if I could turn the clock back I would most certainly arrange Lasting Powers of

Attorney for both Property & Finance and Health & Welfare prior to Norman falling ill. These papers take at least six weeks to register and need to be thought about carefully. Had these papers been in place, I am confident of the following:-

Norman's Financial Advisor would not have been appointed Financial Attorney and my appointment as Attorney would not have been compromised. My stress levels would have been reduced significantly

I believe the Health & Welfare LPA would have ensured my voice being heard and I could have saved Norman from the stress and torment of being subjected to so many mental capacity tests. It is soul destroying trying to care for someone when as far as the NHS is concerned you have "no voice"

It did not take Kevin and I long to instruct a solicitor to raise these documents for each of us and they currently sit at the solicitor's office so we are prepared should either one of us fall ill or have an accident.

4. NHS Continuing Healthcare

NHS Continuing Healthcare is often in the news at the moment. If you are found eligible your care costs will be paid for by the NHS. However if you are not eligible and you have funds over the limit, you will have to pay for your own care costs which may result in the need to sell your property. There are several laws governing this together with case law.

I touched on NHS Continuing Healthcare in Chapter 3 as Norman had to be assessed as part of the discharge procedure from the neurological nursing home. He had been found not to be eligible which, at the time, surprised me as his care needs to cope with his disabilities and illnesses were so great, but my only concern at that time was to achieve his discharge.

Once home, apart from receiving a letter confirming ineligibility, we had no further contact with the Continuing Healthcare team, despite being told that Norman would be reassessed at home within six months. At the time, although a few people had murmured that Norman should be funded I did not for one moment believe that the NHS would not comply with the law or act unprofessionally, nor did I realise that I should become an expert in the field of NHS Continuing Healthcare before attending any meetings. I trusted their integrity and knowledge implicitly.

However, whilst obtaining probate after Norman's death, my own financial planners asked why he had paid for his own care as they believed he should have been funded. I took a little convincing because I was still trusting of the NHS and so my Financial Advisors pointed me to a specialist in Continuing Healthcare who, in turn, directed me to a video on the internet. The specialists I spoke to advised me that, in their opinion, Norman's case was not even a "border line" case; he was well within the limits for eligibility and funding. The more I researched the more I understood what they were saying.

My principled-self erupted to the surface yet again. How dare they (the NHS)?! It was Norman's human right to be funded. As a director of his own company, Norman had paid more NI than most people. How many more people is the NHS unjustly refusing eligibility? How dare the NHS place themselves above the law? Yes, you have guessed it, another fight was about to begin but, yet again, I had no idea how long and time-consuming this fight was going to be. Many families, understandably, are exhausted by the arduous NHS Complaints procedure and give in – not me, I was in there for the long haul! One thing that I did learn very quickly though was to write my comments/observations down as too often verbal comments were twisted and contorted which resulted in too much time being spent on trying to "straighten" the twists rather than on the important and pertinent points.

August 2015 I sent a letter to the CCG who had dealt with Norman's case and had to chase for a reply several times. To be fair this letter was outside the review period but, knowing, they were in the wrong for not reassessing Norman's case at home, the CCG offered to compile a "Retrospective Review" for the period he was at home backdated to the date of discharge. After a further 20 months (yep one year, eight months), I was invited to a panel hearing.

On arrival, I was told that I had 30 minutes to speak at which time I would be asked to leave and their meeting would commence. Having not been informed of this prior to the meeting, I was unprepared. It is fair to say that I "babbled" a bit. Norman was found to be eligible from 1st April 2015 to his date of death in May 2015 but not eligible from 1st April 2014 to 31st March 2015. This, for me, was totally illogical. Despite there not being a medical emergency Norman was not eligible one minute to midnight 31st March 2015 but was eligible at one minute past midnight 1st April 2015. I submitted the paperwork to the NHS Ombudsman who spoke to me three months later saying that they are very sorry but cannot progress my complaint because I have not exhausted the NHS complaints procedure and told me to send another letter to the relevant CCG. The Ombudsman also said that I had to give them the chance to sort this out locally and that I would not be back to the Ombudsman. Picking up on this point, I asked why and she realised that perhaps she had said too much and replied "Well, put it this way, if you come back your complaint will be against the NHS not the local CCG." I sent a further letter as the Ombudsman suggested and a further meeting was arranged with the CCG during which I was told that there were a lot of worrying issues in Norman's case and it was suggested that I take the case to an "Independent Review Panel".

It took a further six months for the local CCG to forward Norman's files to the NHS but eventually an Independent Review Panel date was arranged for February 2018 (ten months after the ombudsman's letter).

Kevin and I travelled by car for three hours to the Independent Review Panel. The Chairman travelled two-and-a-half hours but, surprisingly, the local CCG did not attend. Their contribution was made via a conference call.

It was an experience attending the panel as they are obviously trained not to show any emotion, so it was like talking to brick walls and for me the most interesting point is that although their bible "The National Framework" refers to case law stating that it must be complied to, the panel were not allowed to discuss this. The panel found that the local CCG had not complied to NHS procedures and said they would notify us in six weeks as to whether or not they found Norman eligible. If Norman is found not to be eligible, we have the right to ask the Health Ombudsman to review the case.

Six weeks to the day, an NHS letter enclosing a copy of the panel's report was delivered through our letterbox. The panel found Norman 100% eligible for NHS Continuing Healthcare from the day we discharged him from the nursing home until the day he died. They also found errors within the local CCG's procedures and recommended that the local CCG review their procedures in order to correct their failures. It has taken 4 ½ years since Norman's first assessment and nearly 3 years since my first formal letter of complaint, but finally:-

Feb 2018 - Far too long but I have won – justice for Norman – albeit very late!